CLINICAL CASE
REPORTING IN
EVIDENCE-BASED MEDICINE

D1490093

CLINICAL CASE REPORTING IN EVIDENCE-BASED MEDICINE

MILOS JENICEK MD
Professor (McMaster University)
Professor Emeritus (Université de Montréal)
Adjunct Professor (McGill University)

Hamilton (Ontario) and Montreal (Quebec)
Canada

Second Edition

ARNOLD

A member of the Hodder Headline Group
LONDON
Co-published in the United States of America by
Oxford University Press Inc., New York

First published in Great Britain in 1999 by
Butterworth-Heinemann, a division of Reed Educational
and Professional Publishing

Second edition published in Great Britain in 2001 by
Arnold, a member of the Hodder Headline Group,
338 Euston Road, London NW1 3BH

http://www.arnoldpublishers.com

Co-published in the United States of America by
Oxford University Press Inc.,
198 Madison Avenue, New York, NY10016
Oxford is a registered trademark of Oxford University Press

© 2001 Milos Jenicek

All rights reserved. No part of this publication may be reproduced or
transmitted in any form or by any means, electronically or mechanically,
including photocopying, recording or any information storage or retrieval
system, without either prior permission in writing from the publisher or a
licence permitting restricted copying. In the United Kingdom such licences
are issued by the Copyright Licensing Agency: 90 Tottenham Court Road,
London W1P 0LP.

Whilst the advice and information in this book are believed to be true and
accurate at the date of going to press, neither the authors nor the publisher
can accept any legal responsibility or liability for any errors or omissions
that may be made. In particular (but without limiting the generality of the
preceding disclaimer) every effort has been made to check drug dosages;
however, it is still possible that errors have been missed. Furthermore,
dosage schedules are constantly being revised and new side-effects
recognized. For these reasons the reader is strongly urged to consult the
drug companies' printed instructions before administering any of the drugs
recommended in this book.

British Library Cataloguing in Publication Data
A catalogue record for this book is available from the British Library

Library of Congress Cataloging-in-Publication Data
A catalog record for this book is available from the Library of Congress

ISBN 0 340 76399 X

1 2 3 4 5 6 7 8 9 10

Publisher: Geoffrey Smaldon
Production Editor: Rada Radojicic
Production Controller: Iain McWilliams

Typeset by J&L Composition Ltd, Filey, North Yorkshire
Printed in Malta by Gutenberg Press Ltd

What do you think about this book? Or any other Arnold title?
Please send your comments to feedback.arnold@hodder.co.uk

'. . . Any patient that goes through the door of this hospital is a potential case report . . .'

Anonymous
(The Montreal General Hospital)

CONTENTS

FOREWORD

William Osler's famous statement: *'The best teaching of medicine is that taught by the patient himself'* should be inscribed on the front door of any institution whose mission it is to train young physicians.

Medical diagnosis is the complex art of recognizing illnesses whose signs and symptoms constantly differ from case to case. This task is made all the more difficult by the patient's subjective description of his or her state of health. Thus, the physician's approach should be based on a meticulously organized analysis inevitably put to the test by the theoretical aspects of the pathology. In addition to this quasi-automated process, the clinician's thoughts should also progress through a series of intuitions, each providing hypotheses to be improved upon or rejected as determined by objective confirmatory elements, most often paraclinical in nature.

This phase of diagnosis, which is related to the theory of forms (Gestalt) used in sensory psychology, is entirely reliant on **clinical experience**, the acquisition of which is extremely time-consuming not only during training but also throughout the physician's professional life.

Clinical experience is in fact based on the **observation of clinical cases**.

All medical training, or at least that in the French tradition, relies on the relationship between three actors: the patient, the student and the teacher. The student is required to write down his observations pertaining to a case. The teacher then examines them in detail and presents a logical solution. Thus, attitudes are inherently learnt, pathological examples are committed to memory, and a reference tool much more effective than a paragraph in a book is obtained to aid in the preparation of diagnostic hypotheses.

However, there are times when a more unusual, deceptive case should be described to a larger group: members of a team in a hospital, participants at a scientific symposium, or even the entire medical profession nationally or internationally by means of a specialized journal.

In all these cases, the goal is the same: to convey a message that interests the audience and which is useful to everyone including future patients of an identical pathology.

This presentation of cases with the aim of focusing the medical profession's attention on the peculiar characteristics of an illness is an art that certain clinicians truly master.

In reality, the art of presenting cases should follow the rules set out in this book. Yet, it is also important to note from the start that there is a continuum between writing the details (in a medical chart) of the examination, diagnosis and the therapeutic follow-up that physicians must provide for each patient, followed by the preparation of a 'case report' which can be submitted to the review committee of a prestigious journal.

In addition to its pedagogical benefits, the presentation of clinical cases has heuristic implications. A case marks the beginning of a series of cases and therefore an epidemiological study. It is also the starting point of physiopathological hypotheses leading to confirmatory experimental studies. Numerous examples of this exist and communicable pathologies are a painful reality that have led to the opening of new nosological chapters stemming from a single case (e.g. AIDS, mad cow disease). Many other examples can also be found in pharmacology (the discovery of sulfonylureas for example), to the point where drug monitoring based on case studies has become a fully fledged discipline. In my area of specialty, endocrinology, it is well known that the fundamental role of the thyroid on all bodily functions was suggested to Kocher by the single observation of a patient who had recently undergone a thyroidectomy.

It is logical that Milos Jenicek, who is interested in teaching clinical research methodology, seeks to help our young colleagues improve their 'clinical case report' writing. Thus, Chapter 5 of this book, 'How to prepare a single case report', is an invaluable tool. This chapter covers everything, from the reasons for a clinical case report, the selection of data and the format of the discussion, to the choice of bibliographical material. It also gives semantic hints.

Milos Jenicek is of the North American school, and more specifically of the Canadian school, which prizes the theorization of medical activity. The notion of clinical epidemiology derives from these approaches and Milos Jenicek has produced a number of works on the topic. In one of these, he tackled a new domain of clinimetrics, a term coined by A.R. Feinstein. In this book, with regards to the relationship between clinical cases, he focuses on 'medical casuistics'. By way of a very clever semiotic analysis, he justifies the transfer of this theological term to the medical field.

Certainly, French medical culture is less avid for new concepts, rating scales and indexes than its North American equivalent, but since the author's background is varied, partly due to numerous teaching assignments in Europe, he seamlessly links together these two approaches.

Therefore, this work, as the author had hoped, *'helps young clinicians communicate clinical observations in a clear, comprehensible and complete manner'*. It is my belief that the result will be even more far-reaching than that. By 'coding' the process, Milos Jenicek provides a successful formula for rigorous analysis and presentation. He stresses, in fact, that *'no matter what the format of the presentation, the beginner will quickly come to realize that the evaluation of a case is actually the first task to accomplish'*.

Thus, we return to clinical teaching. By formalizing information recording, the reasoning process is supported. To paraphrase Boileau, *'that which is well designed can be clearly stated'*, and it is not by chance that the writing of a book, thesis or review has become a step in the thought pattern of the student. In addition, the emphasis placed on the quality of medical record keeping today will gradually lead to the inclusion of this parameter in the evaluation of physicians' activities.

The training of future evaluators according to a reading scale for documents that are presented to them is a final practical and positive result of this book.

RENÉ MORNEX
Professor Emeritus
Claude Bernard University
Corresponding member of the
French Academy of Medicine

PREFACE

With the rise of strong clinical research in this century, case reports have been treated with ambivalence. On the one hand, serious researchers know that case reports fall far short in terms of scientific credibility. They cannot match the decisiveness of randomized controlled trials, the power of large cohort studies, or the elegance of case control studies in the right hands. On the other hand, physicians in practice like them. Clinicians prefer to learn from individual cases, either their own or a colleague's, and published case reports retain a strong connection with their simpler cousins, the case descriptions presented at the bedside or discussed over lunch.

In this book, Milos Jenicek helps us understand the place of case reports in medicine, especially the *'special cases that advance the knowledge, research and practice of medicine'*. He writes mainly about the cases that are described to a broad audience in journal articles and not about case reporting to local colleagues at the bedside. He recognizes that case reports are a large and neglected part of the medical literature and helps to raise their level of quality.

Case reports have long been familiar elements of medical journals and they remain so. During the period 1946–1976, single case reports comprised 13 per cent of articles in leading medical journals, and 38 per cent of articles were of ten or fewer patients and thus, for scientific purposes, were like single case reports. And case reports, in one form or another, are still a regular feature of major clinical journals today, albeit in various forms. *The Lancet* publishes case reports under just that heading in nearly every issue and takes great pains to make the cases interesting and instructive, even though most are not so rare as to be first reports. Other journals, such as *The New England Journal of Medicine* and *Annals of Internal Medicine*, have taken to publishing full research articles in their Brief Reports sections which were formerly reserved for case reports, but continue to publish accounts of single cases as letters – and sometimes even as original articles. *The New England Journal of Medicine* also uses individual cases to teach clinical medicine through its series Clinical Problem Solving. The less widely circulated peer reviewed journals, which comprise more of the world's medical journals, continue to publish single case reports, as they always have.

Can the enduring popularity of case reports be justified on scientific grounds ? After all, they can offer no credible evidence on the rate of clinical events, a central element in studies of the natural history of disease. And, because they include no comparison (control) group, they are severely limited as a way of understanding risk factors and causes of disease, and the effectiveness of therapeutic or preventive interventions.

But case reports do serve other purposes, also important to scientific progress. What can they do that large, controlled studies cannot?

Case reports are the only source of information on rare events. If one has a patient in the office with an unusual symptom – perhaps a potential drug reaction – where else can one turn for guidance, however limited ? Case reports are also a rich source of hypotheses. All that we know about clinical HIV infection or toxic shock syndrome began with observations of individual cases. Case reports can be a vehicle for teaching clinical medicine. For example, many physicians may have forgotten what they learned in medical school about patent ductus arteriosus and find in a properly presented case an opportunity to review cardiac physiology, even if the case itself is not unique. And yes, case reports can entertain. The former editor of the *British Medical Journal*, Steven Lock, pointed out that *'scientific journals have several functions: to inform, instruct, comment and, possibly, amuse'* in order to maintain a strong place in the lives of busy clinicians. For this reason, when my wife and I were editors of *Annals of Internal Medicine* we decided to publish a case report of a man and his dog, both stricken with histoplasmosis while he was chopping a rotten log, complete with chest radiographs of both patients.

Case reports are most valuable as part of a comprehensive database of other case reports, which can be searched when needed. Finding the case report one wants when one needs it is far more feasible now that Medline searching is free to users and the World Wide Web has made literature searching widely available throughout the world. After all, few clinicians read any one journal, and by definition they are unlikely to find in it information about the specific rare event that they need to know about.

Milos Jenicek has written a comprehensive book about case reports: what makes them useful, how they fit into the totality of scientific evidence, and how they should be described in writing. A few other scholars have written chapters and articles about case reports, describing their components and style, and what editors and reviewers looks for in the ones they publish. Dr Jenicek's book includes these elements in greater depth, but he has also gone a step further. He places case reports in the context of modern clinical science by establishing connections between single case reports, case series and more elaborate and powerful studies, such as cohort and case control studies and clinical trials.

So case reports are not on the fringe of science and clinical practice, as they are sometimes believed to be. They deserve serious, scholarly consideration. Dr Jenicek has given them the attention they deserve.

ROBERT H. FLETCHER
Professor
Harvard Medical School
and Harvard School of Public Health

Introductory comments: objectives and contents of this book

As long as medicine exists, physicians will share their clinical case experiences with their colleagues. However, if the unique, the exceptional and the extraordinary are not properly recorded, a good portion of the progress achieved in terms of patient care, originality, innovation, and enrichment of medical thinking will be lost, possibly forever.

The objective of this brief guide is to help young clinicians understand and prepare meaningful clinical case reports.

Clinicians have always recounted to their peers the circumstances, patient outcomes and consequences of the cases they have encountered. This is and will always be a powerful means of learning and further developing the practice of medicine.

Clinical cases are presented everywhere: on hospital floors, on daily ward rounds and on grand rounds, as well as in seminars, in meetings, in the medical press and at conventions. Wherever reports of this type are made, the initial physician–patient interaction marks the beginning of the acquisition of medical knowledge and of the professional and scientific retelling of lived experience.

A process of such importance cannot rely solely on gut feelings and on the natural intelligence of current and forthcoming generations. Unfortunately, our medical forefathers often played this trick on us. In reality, the form and content or 'direction' of case reporting must be learnt like anything else. And herein lies the purpose of this book.

The reader will be presented with nine chapters, as outlined below.

In the first chapter, the concept and objectives of modern medical casuistics, i.e. the recording and study of cases of disease[1], will be explained.

In the second chapter, the reader will find an overview of the Evidence-Based Medicine and the place of clinical case reports in this field.

In the third, the reader will see that medical casuistics or clinical case reporting is simply a part of a wider field of case studies in human sciences and a current end-product of a long history of thinking in the health, social and business sciences. In fact, clinical case reporting can be considered a component of the rapidly developing qualitative research field, and therefore complements its basic fundamental clinical, bedside clinical and field epidemiological quantitative constituents.

In the fourth, routine case reporting methodology is outlined.

In the fifth chapter, step by step instructions cover the preparation of a good clinical case report, mainly for the purpose of publication in the medical press.

In the sixth, basic principles, methods and techniques of clinical case reporting are further illustrated using an annotated example of a good clinical case report as published recently in a medical journal. This chapter will demonstrate that an increasing number of presentations already effectively follow the guidelines set forth in this book.

The seventh chapter covers case series reports – the description and analysis of more than one case.

The eighth chapter shows briefly what more can be done in medical research based on single cases or case series.

The ninth chapter summarizes the major points of the previous chapters and offers strategic tips for future clinical practice and research.

Many readers might ask why a clinical epidemiologist would tackle the area of clinical case reporting. There are two reasons for this. The first is that accurate descriptions of clinical cases now rely heavily on clinical epidemiology and clinimetrics (measurement and classification of clinical observations). The second is that, at the

How this book should be read:

- You do not have an immediate opportunity to get a balanced view of what Evidence-Based Medicine is today and wonder if and how clinical case reporting fits into this stimulating domain. Read Chapter 2.
- If you have never done a routine clinical case report, you have to do it right now and if nobody told you how, because "you are clever enough, you will figure it out, just look how obvious it is", read Chapter 4.
- If you are a busy intern or resident wanting to master only the essential steps of preparing a publication oriented clinical case report, read Chapter 5.
- If you are looking for a concrete example of a well-prepared published case, read Chapter 6.
- If you have a curious mind and wish to know what more research might be done on the basis of a single case or case series, read Chapter 8.
- If you are a clinical teacher or an intellectual luminary who feels it necessary to possess a broad knowledge of everything, read this book from cover to cover.

moment, when index cases of some new or otherwise relevant clinical phenomena are observed, elucidated and described, new hypotheses arise and further causal, treatment or prognostic research ideas are triggered.

We have learnt a great deal about the methodology required to adequately describe disease occurrence, to illustrate its cases, to demonstrate the most effective, efficient and efficacious treatment, to understand disease prognosis, to produce the best research synthesis and to make complex decisions in practice. However, we have not yet invested a similar effort in the area of clinical case reporting, the building block of all of these elements.

There are two levels of clinical case reporting. Routine cases are reported in day to day ward or office practice. This is of special interest to those in clinical service. Special cases that advance the knowledge, research and practice of medicine are also reported. This book focuses mainly on the latter.

Presently, clinical case reporting appears to be another necessary training tool for our graduate students in clinical epidemiology.

Is this subject entirely new? Not exactly. It is in some way a product of the ebb and flow of medicine between the Old and New Worlds. In the past century, many North American, Asian and African physicians travelled to Germany and France to master the thinking and workings of medicine at that time. They met such people as Pierre-Charles Alexandre Louis (1787–1872) who helped transform medicine into a science based on observation by rigorously following up on and systematically recording the vital functions of his patients. He also compiled other clinical observations, thus unknowingly becoming one of the forefathers of clinical epidemiology. Pinel, Laënnec, Bichat, Corvisart and Martinet were among those who personified the French school of medicine that focused on the detailed recording of history, disease manifestations and autopsies. Soon after, the German and Austrian schools (led by Mueller, Rokitanski and Skoda, among others) served as training grounds for North American physicians. Thus, William Osler was able to reiterate the importance of history and clinical examinations as a fundamental part of case recording and reports[2]. Generations have now elapsed since these migrations of ideas and experiences between the Old and the New Worlds.

Today, **evidence-based medicine**[3], born from Canadian experience and innovation, reverses the tide of medical reasoning and thinking and subjects it to the test of time. Since evidence-based medicine makes use of the most complete information available on diagnostic methods, disease occurrence and effectiveness of prevention or treatment, complete evidence from clinical cases must be provided.

It is important to realize that, before evidence of aetiology or treatment effectiveness is established, evidence of cases and their occurrence is required. Is this possible without a proper clinical case reporting methodology? Definitely not. Very occasionally, methodologically remarkable proofs of aetiology or treatment effectiveness are based only on 'mirages' of cases; they should not be. **Cases themselves are and must be the first line of evidence**.

The reader will benefit from an *a priori* knowledge of clinical epidemiology and clinimetrics. Although this monograph explains a few of the basic concepts of these fields, it is not a true substitute for *ad hoc* textbooks entirely devoted to them. This book does, however, strive to be accessible subsequent or parallel reading for the novice, and an essential tool for the busy clinician.

As William Makepeace Thackeray once said, *'the two most engaging powers of an author are to make new things familiar and familiar things new'*. This text tries to do both. It is based largely on my last work in French[4], which was perhaps the first to focus on today's modern medical casuistics. However, recent advances in clinical sciences compelled me to offer this more complete and updated message.

A small army of highly qualified and experienced friends and colleagues have reviewed and greatly improved my work: Carol-Ann Oldbury from the Montérégie Public Health Directorate (word processing and general text review), Jacques Cadieux of the Université de Montréal (infographics), Nicole Kinney of Lingua-max (literary and stylistic review), Drs Karl Weiss and Denise Ouellette of the Maisonneuve-Rosemont Hospital (medicine and surgery), Zorana Prelevic of the McGill University Health Centre (psychiatry), Gordon Guyatt of the McMaster University (*n*-of-1 clinical trials), Stephen Walter of the McMaster University and Muin Khoury of the Centers for Disease Control and Prevention in Atlanta, GA (genetic epidemiology); and Ann McKibbon, Cindy Walker-Dilks and Angela Eady of the McMaster University Health Information Research Unit (general readability review). All these people made this book possible and I am grateful to them.

REFERENCES

1. *Miller-Keane Encyclopedia & Dictionary of Medicine, Nursing & Allied Health*, 6th Edition. Philadelphia: WB Saunders, 1997.
2. Walker HK. The origins of the history and physical examination, pp. 22–28 in: *Clinical Methods. The History, Physical, and Laboratory Examination*, 3rd Edition. Edited by HK Walker, WD Wall and JW Hurst. Boston: Butterworths, 1988.
3. Sackett DL, Richardson WS, Rosenberg W, Haynes B. *Evidence-Based Medicine. How to Practice and Teach EBM*. New York: Churchill Livingstone, 1997.
4. Jenicek M. *Casuistique Médicale. Bien Présenter un Cas Clinique. (Medical Casuistics. Presenting a Clinical Case Well.)* St Hyacinthe and Paris: Edisem and Maloine, 1997.

CHAPTER 1

The importance
of modern case
reporting or
medical
casuistics

CHAPTER 1

For many, a clinical report focused on an isolated case means nothing. In reality, if our peers do not select a relevant topic and present it properly, the medical community barely stifles a yawn.

The importance of modern case reporting or medical casuistics

1.1 CASE REPORTING AS A FIELD OF DISSENT

Recently, a British psychiatry resident complained in a Letter to the Editor of a journal[1]: *'after reading the case report "Suspicion of somatoform disorder in undiagnosed tabes dorsalis[2]" I found myself puzzled as to what I should learn from it. Tabes dorsalis is adequately described in most of the standard textbooks, and the fact that a psychiatric assessment was solicited before the investigation had confirmed the diagnosis, seems a curious reason for a case report, particularly such a long one. Good case reports are instructive and illuminating. Could I make a plea that, in view of the burgeoning numbers of case reports, only those which present truly novel observations be selected for publication?'.* (N.B. The Editor defended the novelty of the observation.)

Was this case report really poorly presented? Was the resident at fault for not learning what he was supposed to? Or was it a little of both?

1.2   CLINICAL CASE REPORTING TODAY

This example shows that clinical case reporting today requires methodologies and selection criteria probably as stringent as that of any other basic or decision-oriented clinical research field.

Since antiquity, physicians have learnt from their more experienced peers, as well as from their own successes and failures. Accurate recounting of clinical experience continues to be essential to the progress of medicine, because it marks the beginning of the longer and increasingly complex process of learning initiated by observations made at the patient's bedside. For example, before the clinical characteristics and epidemiology of the Ebola virus-related haemorrhagic fever were established, the first cases had to be correctly described. The analysis and subsequent synthesis of this new problem only occurred once this was done.

An interesting case, such as an unusual cerebral embolism or mycotic infection may become an 'index case', thus launching a search for similar occurrences and helping to determine the importance of frequency in similar cases within communities of interest. These steps may lead to the formulation of a hypothesis concerning the new diagnostic entity, its possible causes and treatment.

Nowadays, medicine is widening its focus and objectives, i.e. to prevent and treat disease, to protect individuals and communities, and to promote the best health possible in as many people as possible. It has replaced its paradigm of art and deterministic science with a paradigm of probabilistic science based on decisions made in uncertain situations.

Basic clinical or laboratory research, which is essentially explanatory, now has a counterpart in decision- and action-oriented 'bedside' clinical research. Clinical epidemiology and biostatistics have quickly become pivotal in this evolution of medicine where a new and better equilibrium has been established for art and science. At the end of such a learning process, the results obtained from observation and experience are reapplied at the starting point, namely, the clinical work for an individual patient and the care provided to communities.

If 'serious' medicine aspires to have its own 'letters of nobility', it should not be forgotten that everything begins with the personal experience of the physician and his patient, at the office or hospital. If this groundwork is not correct, the study of disease occurrence, aetiological research and clinical trials are worth very little. Similarly, medical intervention is of little value if there is poor handling of individual cases of the disease in question.

A resident on night call has admitted a new patient. He performs a complete work-up, gives his 'impression' of the major clues leading to the differential diagnosis and orders a treatment plan to 'stabilize' the patient. The next morning, the resident has to present this new case to his or her peers. If particularly interesting, the 'case' may be presented on floor rounds or grand rounds or ultimately reported in the medical press. However, floor or grand presentations and clinical case reporting in the medical press must abide by the specific rules detailed in the following chapters.

There are three levels of case reporting, each with different goals.

1. **Floor or daily ward presentations** often include all cases indiscriminately. These types of reports serve administrative purposes. They also ensure continuity and completeness of care.
2. Only selected cases are presented on **rounds.** The cases may be scientifically relevant but the reports themselves generally strive to ensure better operation of in-house work.
3. **Clinical case reports in the medical press** represent (or should represent) a scientific endeavour comparable to other observational or experimental research projects.

This book focuses mainly on the principles, methods and techniques of special clinical case presentations produced for the medical press. Compared to the more clearly established standards of in-house presentations, written clinical case reporting requires the mastery of additional rules (as detailed in Chapter 5) leading to clear, effective, comprehensible and complete presentations. Any intern or resident should follow these rules.

Yet we tend to derive our attitudes, knowledge, skills and experience from various sets of observations based on the current standards of clinical epidemiology. We know what to do with repeated observations and experience. However, do we know equally well how to study an 'individual' and how to share such an experience with others? Do we need more specific training in this area?

Responsible clinical researchers manage to publish two or three original papers in a year. In contrast, practising clinicians must, almost immediately, discuss their experiences with individual patients, either orally or in writing. If these practising clinicians prepare their reports correctly, and this book aims to help them achieve this goal, their contributions should be even more significant to the advancement of our medical wisdom.

Well-selected and adequately presented clinical cases are an important tool in the acquisition and comprehension of new information. Reports on the first cases of toxic shock syndrome or necrotizing fasciitis led to the study of series of such cases, and ultimately to the understanding of their causes and treatment.

Clinical case reporting in the medical press remains a controversial topic. However, if the report is good, its publication should be encouraged without hesitation[3-5].

Not so long ago, journals as distinguished as *Cancer* often simply discarded clinical case reports. Such decisions may have been motivated by the desire to include only preferred topics that the Editors had deemed 'absolute priorities'. These decisions might also have been made to avoid the ever-increasing flood of sometimes questionable information. How then is particularly bad reporting to be controlled?

Chew[6] recently analysed the fate of clinical case reports submitted to the *American Journal of Roentgenology*. Only one in five (20 per cent) reports submitted was effectively published.

However, it should be noted that there are many other reputed journals whose Editors encourage the publication of well-selected, relevant and impeccably presented cases. Such articles are an integral part of the medical culture since they enrich professional experience and lead to better clinical reasoning, often triggering 'more serious' research.

Case Records of the Massachusetts General Hospital in *The New England Journal of Medicine* or Clinical Reports in *The Lancet*, or Case Studies in *The Canadian Medical Association Journal*, or even issues of the *Journal of Obstetrics and Gynecology* devoted to special clinical cases, are just a few illustrations of these editorial policies.

1.3 CONTEMPORARY DEVELOPMENTS IN CLINICAL CASE REPORTING

The modern clinical case report was made possible by the recent development of clinical epidemiology[7–12], and of clinimetrics[9,13,14] in particular.

> Any study of multiple cases must derive from the study of one individual case. The study of both individual and multiple cases requires adequate gathering of clinical data, hardening of soft data, conversion of data into clinical information, appropriate reproduction of the pathway from clinical observation to diagnosis, well-structured descriptions of the natural history and of the natural and clinical course of the disease, clear pictures of the gradient and spectrum of the pathology under study, and the selection of eloquent paraclinical data.
>
> A statement highlighting the pragmatic questions to be answered by a case study and the operational results expected from such an endeavour has quickly become a requirement.

At present, we are inspired by the development and the results of research in human biology and pathology, by decision-oriented clinical research based on clinical epidemiology and biostatistics, and by the results of an evidence-based approach in medicine.

Individual case studies must catch up with other fields of medical research in their observational and analytical methodology, as well as in their interpretation and presentation.

The clinical case paradigm has become more defined and structured. Clinical epidemiology provides it with the tools necessary to make clinical case experience both operational and beneficial for the patient, and useful for the physician.

Today, general practitioners and specialists in training acquire an increasingly adequate clinical attitude, knowledge and set of skills. They also learn how to better read, interpret and integrate into their practice the results of original studies and papers[15-30]. Unfortunately, they do not always know how to prepare and present a clinical case[31] and how to retain the most important and useful information for their future practice.

In fact, we have searched in vain in the literature for a monograph devoted to clinical case reporting in terms of medical casuistics.

Hospital rounds often focus on the basics of the pathology, diagnosis and treatment[32] of relevant cases. However, case presentations are more involved than that. They represent an exercise in the organization of thought, in the acquisition of relevant clinical and paraclinical information, and in the making of correct clinical decisions.

Petrusa and Weiss[33] suggest that every physician in training should prepare and present at least one acceptable clinical case in terms of form and content.

The design and presentation of a clinical case report are not only important teaching tools. Supported by clinimetrics, they lead the authors of the reports towards other fields of clinical research. The following chapters outline the ideas and elements that constitute a structured approach to the work-up and presentation of clinical cases.

Are these details necessary? Definitely. Until now, only two textbooks on epidemiology have briefly touched upon the topic of desirable contents of case reports[34,35]. Other contributions to the field focus more on structure and style than on what should be in a report and what should be left out. None of these sources provides indications concerning the preparation, content and architecture of a case report for publication. Chapter 5 will meet this objective.

Despite the humble background of clinical case presentations, reporting unique experiences in comparison with aetiologic research or clinical trials will always remain a powerful aid in generating research and clinical experience.

REFERENCES

1. Pearson R. Case report criticism. (Correspondence) *Br J Psychiatry*, 1992; **160**: 280.
2. Fichtner CG, Weddington WW. Suspicion of somatoform disorder in undiagnosed tabes dorsalis. *Br J Psychiatry*,1991; **159**: 573–5.
3. Soffer A. Case reports in the Archives of Internal Medicine. *Arch Intern Med*,1976; **136**: 1090.
4. Nahum AM. The clinical case report: 'Pot boiler' or scientific literature? *Head & Neck Surg*,1979; **1**: 291–2.
5. Simpson RJ Jr, Griggs TR. Case reports and medical progress. *Persp Biol Med*,1985; **28**: 402–6.
6. Chew FS. Fate of manuscripts rejected for publication in the AJR. *AJR*,1991; **156**: 627–32.
7. Fletcher RH, Fletcher SW, Wagner EH. *Clinical Epidemiology – The Essentials.* Baltimore and London: Williams and Wilkins, 1982 (3rd Edition: 1996).
8. Jenicek M, Cléroux R. *Épidémiologie. Principes, techniques, applications. (Epidemiology. Principles, Techniques, Applications.)* St Hyacinthe and Paris: Edisem and Maloine,1982 (see Chapter 14).
9. Jenicek M, Cléroux R. *Épidémiologie clinique. Clinimétrie. (Clinical Epidemiology. Clinimetrics.)* St Hyacinthe and Paris: Edisem and Maloine, 1985.
10. Feinstein AR. *Clinical Epidemiology. The Architecture of Clinical Research.* Philadelphia: WB Saunders,1985.
11. Sackett DL, Haynes RB, Tugwell PX. *Clinical Epidemiology: A Basic Science for Clinical Practice.* Boston: Little, Brown, 1984.
12. Jenicek M. *Epidemiology. The Logic of Modern Medicine.* Montreal: Epimed International, 1995.
13. Feinstein AR. An additional basic science for clinical medicine: IV. The development of clinimetrics. *Ann Intern Med*,1983; **99**: 843–8.
14. Feinstein AR. *Clinimetrics.* New Haven: Yale University Press, 1987.
15. Gehlbach SH, Bobula JA, Dickinson JC. Teaching residents to read medical literature. *J Med Educ*,1980; **55**: 362–5.
16. Oxman AD, Sackett DL, Guyatt GH for the Evidence-Based Medicine Working Group. Users' guides to the medical literature. I. How to get started. *JAMA*,1993; **270:** 2093–5.
17. Guyatt GH, Sackett DL, Cook DJ for the Evidence-Based Medicine Working Group. Users' guides to the medical literature. II. How to use an article about therapy or prevention: A. Are the results valid? *JAMA*,1993; **270**: 2598–601;

B. What were the results and will they help me in caring for my patients? *JAMA*,1994; **271**: 59–63.

18. Jeaschke R, Guyatt G, Sackett DL for the Evidence-Based Medicine Working Group. Users' guides to the medical literature. III. How to use an article about a diagnostic test: A. Are the results of the study valid? *JAMA*,1994; **271**: 389–91; B. What are the results and will they help me in caring for my patients? *JAMA*,1994; **271**: 703–7.

19. Levine M, Walter S, Lee H, Haines T, Holbrook A, Moyer V for the Evidence-Based Medicine Working Group. Users' guides to the medical literature. IV. How to use an article about harm. *JAMA*,1994; **271**: 1615–9.

20. Laupacis A, Wells G, Richardson S, Tugwell P for the Evidence-Based Medicine Working Group. Users' guides to the medical literature. V. How to use an article about prognosis. *JAMA*,1994; **272**: 234–7.

21. Oxman AD, Cook DJ, Guyatt GH for the Evidence-Based Medicine Working Group. Users' guides to the medical literature. VI. How to use an overview. *JAMA*,1994; **272**: 1367–71.

22. Richardson SW, Destsky AS for the Evidence-Based Medicine Working Group. User's guides to the medical literature. VII. How to use a clinical decision analysis: A. Are the results of the study valid? *JAMA*,1995; **273**; 1292–5; B. What are the results and will they help me in caring for my patients? *JAMA*,1995; **273**: 1610–3.

23. Hayward RSA, Wilson MC, Tunis SR, Bass EB, Guyatt G for the Evidence-Based Medicine Working Group. Users' guides to the medical literature. VIII. How to use clinical practice guidelines: A. Are the recommendations valid? *JAMA*,1995; **274**: 570–4.

24. Wilson MC, Hayward SA, Tunis SR, Bass EB, Guyatt G for the Evidence-Based Medicine Working Group. Users' guides to the medical literature. VIII. How to use clinical practice guidelines: B. What are the recommendations and will they help you in caring for your patients? *JAMA*,1995; **274**: 1630–2.

25. Guyatt GH, Sackett DL, Sinclair JC, Hayward R, Cook DJ, Cook RJ for the Evidence-Based Medicine Working Group. Users' guides to the medical literature. IX. A method for grading health care recommendations. *JAMA*, 1995; **274**: 1800–4.

26. Naylor CD, Guyatt GH, for the Evidence-Based Medicine Working Group. Users' guides to the medical literature. X. How to use an article reporting variations in the outcomes of health services. *JAMA*,1996; **275**: 554–8.

27. Naylor CD, Guyatt GH for the Evidence-Based Medicine Working Group. Users' guides to the medical literature. XI. How to use an article about a clinical utilization review. *JAMA*,1996; **275**: 1435–9.

28. Guyatt GH, Naylor CD, Juniper E, Heyland DK, Jaeschke R, Cook DJ for the Evidence-Based Medicine Working Group. Users' guides to the medical literature. XII. How to use articles about health-related quality of life. *JAMA*,1997; **277**: 1232–7.

29. Drummond MF, Richardson SW, O'Brien BJ, Levine M, Heyland D for the Evidence-Based Medicine Working Group. Users' guides to the medical literature. XIII. How to use an article on economic analysis of clinical practice: A. Are the results of the study valid? *JAMA*,1997; **277**: 1552–7.

30. O'Brien BJ, Heyland D, Richardson WS, Levine M, Drummond MF for the Evidence-Based Medicine Working Group. Users' guides to the medical literature. XIII. How to use an article on economic analysis of clinical practice: B. What are the results and will they help me in caring for my patients? *JAMA*,1997; **277**: 1802–6.

31. Huston P, Squires BP. Case reports: Information for authors and peer reviewers. *CMAJ*,1996; **154**: 43–4.

32. Loschen EL. The resident conference: A method to enhance academic intensity. *J Med Educ*,1980; **55**: 209–10.

33. Petrusa ER, Weiss GB. Writing case reports: An educationally valuable experience for house officers. *J Med Educ*,1982; **57**: 415–7.

34. Fletcher RH, Fletcher SW and Wagner EH. Case reports (Chapter 10), pp. 208–211 in: *Clinical Epidemiology. The Essentials*, 3rd Edition. Baltimore: Williams & Wilkins, 1996.

35. Jenicek M. General requirements of good case studies (Chapter 5, Section 5.2.4), pp. 135–136 in: *Epidemiology. The Logic of Modern Medicine*. Montreal: Epimed International, 1995.

Evidence-based medicine: a niche for clinical case reports. The role of case reports in EBM

CHAPTER 2

Evidence-based medicine: a niche for clinical case reports. The role of case reports in EBM

2.1 INTRODUCTORY REMARKS

In true Hippocratic fashion, physicians always tried to provide their patients with the best possible care. In order to meet this goal, evidence on which decisions could be based was needed. Thus, clinical case observation and reporting was born.

- Are clinical case reports worthy of attention? Do they really offer valuable and sufficient evidence for medical decision-making in prevention, clinical care, health programs and policies?
- How do clinical case reports fit into the new and increasingly popular concept and practice of evidence-based medicine (EBM)?
- What is evidence-based medicine?

In medicine and all other health sciences, there is a constant search for the **best evidence** in an effort to prevent or cure physical, mental or social ailments and to promote the best possible health. What method most easily diagnoses a problem? What is the most effective treatment? What allows us to develop the most accurate prognosis and to choose an appropriate course of action for patient outcomes? What should we tell patients to help them lead as productive and happy a life as possible? In the past, religious faith was sufficient to give direction to individuals and communities. Today, more is needed.

Evidence of what is good for mankind shifted first from personal and collective experiences to **basic sciences**. Laboratories were supposed to provide all the answers. Pathology, physiology, biochemistry or genetics were the key to success. More recently, **new technologies** in diagnostic imagery, development of drugs, surgery, or information have led to important advances. Lately such fundamental research has been enhanced by 'bedside clinical research'. Thus, a methodology of clinical and public health decisions based on evidence, probability, uncertainty, economic, social, cultural, political and ethical considerations was established from 'evidence' coming from the other side of the laboratory door.

Epidemiology and biostatistics gave the health sciences reassuring definitions, **quantitative information** and their interpretation. In other fields, such as psychology, psychiatry and nursing, a desire to understand better what was 'behind and beside the numbers' led to the development and use of **qualitative research**. Today, clinical reporting reflects the new tendency to integrate both quantitative and qualitative research in our understanding of health and disease.

Observing and reporting clinical cases was a type of first line evidence seemingly as old as medicine itself. These activities led clinicians to perform more in-depth research and to understand health problems better. They also served as a first line of evidence in public health: an unusual occurrence of a disease is often signalled by one or more index cases which must be properly described and understood before a detailed investigation of a disease outbreak or other high occurrence is attempted. Other 'evidence' had also been gathered from occurrence studies, aetiological research, clinical trials, field epidemiological intelligence and intervention, prognostic studies, risk and disease surveillance.

The identification of the best evidence from among all these sources and the use of this evidence to make medical decisions gradually became more structured and organized. The process was even given an attractive new name: **evidence-based medicine** or **EBM**[1]. Clinical case reports became a major component of this field.

2.2 HISTORICAL CONTEXT OF EVIDENCE-BASED MEDICINE

Until the mid 19th century, personal and peer experience were practically the only sources of 'evidence', until 'evidence' was split into more clearly defined categories.

One such source of evidence was laboratory studies and data leading to a better understanding of the anatomical–pathological mechanisms of disease, pharmacodynamics and body responses to risk factors, exposure and therapeutic interventions. French, German and Austrian medicine excelled in this area.

The second source of evidence was derived from the increasingly rigorous definition, gathering, analysis, and interpretation of numerical information from demography, public health and clinical medicine. British and North American contributions were considerable here. Such innovative works as Morris' *Uses of Epidemiology*[2] or MacMahon and Pugh's *Epidemiology*[3] impressed and influenced us.

In addition, the North American way of thinking in business, finances, military operations, social sciences, medicine and other health-related fields, brought with it the paradigm of working and making decisions based on probability, uncertainty and incomplete information. The shift from deterministic to probabilistic medicine continued to gain strength.

Chinese, Japanese and Korean medicines maintained and developed systems that combined the best of 'Western' and traditional Asian medicines, paving the way for a better understanding and evaluation of 'alternative' medicines.

The fundamental methodology of drawing information from the case itself about the disease, its aetiology and ways to control it emerged from the public health field. This is also known as 'shoe leather' epidemiology.

Clinical epidemiology[4-8], born in the 1970s and 1980s was somewhat the opposite of the classical approach[9,10]: It used epidemiological information obtained from the study of groups of patients and the community to make the best possible bedside decisions for an individual patient.

Especially in the latter area, we rapidly came to realize that an acceptable quantity of data was usable only if the quality of data was satisfactory. Thus, clinimetrics[11,12] was created to establish the rules of 'quality production, use and control' in medicine.

Finally, we became increasingly interested in the efficaciousness (in model or ideal conditions), effectiveness (under current conditions) and efficiency (at what price) of our clinical and preventive practices.

Ideally, evidence-based medicine should take into account all these historical sources and needs for 'evidence' and in fact, if practised properly, it does.

2.3 WHAT IS 'EVIDENCE'?

According to Webster's Dictionary[13], 'evidence' can be defined as follows:

- Any ground or reason for knowledge or certitude in knowledge.
- Proof, whether immediate or derived by inference.

CLINICAL CASE REPORTING

- A fact or body of facts on which a proof, belief, or judgement is based.
- In law: That by means of which a fact is established: distinguished from *proof*, which is the result of *evidence*, and *testimony*, which is evidence given orally.

Hence, for our purposes, 'evidence' may be seen as:

- Any data or information, whether solid or weak, obtained through experience, observational research or experimental work (trials). This data or information must be relevant either to the understanding of the problem (case) or to the clinical decisions (diagnostic, therapeutic or care-oriented) made about the case.

For Auclair[14], '... *to qualify as a basis for medicine, evidence should have two characteristics that together are necessary and sufficient: it should consist of an observation that has been assessed as valid by experts knowledgeable in the field, and it should impart such a degree of probability on the* (subjective) *hypothesis that it is preferable that we act on it.* ...'

A randomized multiple blind controlled clinical trial may conceptually provide the best cause–effect (treatment–cure) evidence. However, this type of study may be unethical, unsuitable or unfeasible, in which case, other evidence must be considered to be better. All practitioners quickly find that they must make decisions based on evidence of variable strength.

If EBM emphasizes working with the 'best' evidence, the concept of 'best' poses a great challenge. In molecular[15,16] or genetic[17] epidemiology, the best evidence may be sought in the subtle understanding of biological components, mechanisms and interactions at the subcellular level or the interacting pathways of genetic and other factors pertaining to disease risk or prognosis. From the conceptual and methodological standpoint in clinical epidemiology, a randomized double blind controlled trial is better evidence that treatment works than a clinical case report or case series report.

In fact, many have established hierarchical classifications of evidence according to its strength[18,19]. Usually, these systems propose five levels of evidence, based on the capacity of different types of studies to establish a cause–effect link between treatment and cure or noxious agents and disease development:

I. Randomized controlled clinical trials.
II. Non-randomized trials or those with high alpha and beta errors.
III. Analytical observational studies.
IV. Multiple time series or place comparisons, uncontrolled experiments.
V. Expert opinions, descriptive occurrence studies, case reports, case series reports.

Most concerns pertaining to this type of classification of evidence are generally centred on the indiscriminate application of 'best evidence' to particular subgroups of patients[20]. In reality, a good cohort or case–control study may be better than a poorly designed, poorly executed and poorly interpreted randomized controlled clinical trial.

By contrast, a simple case series report of *Pneumocystis carinii* in homosexual men, index case reports of acquired immunodeficiency syndrome or a formulation of viral aetiology of AIDS based on an associative reasoning compared with hepatitis B are examples[14] where such 'low level evidences' are good enough to change and expand follow-up of patients, formulate a new disease entity or consider its infectiousness and mode of transmission.

In the case of a new topic, single case reports are often the only evidence available in the absence of more important clinical trials. For example, if a new gene therapy is first tested at an annual cost of $100,000 per person, notwithstanding ethical considerations and the complexity of producing the treatment modality, a *lege artis* clinical trial might not be possible for some time.

In this sense, the evidence that emerges from clinical case reports must be considered as potentially sufficient without necessarily being the 'best'. However, clinical case reports are clearly always the first line of evidence at a patient's bedside!

Evidence from original studies is rarely homogeneous in the literature and contradictory results as evidence can be produced.

By necessity then, the second source of evidence is a 'study of studies' i.e. meta-analysis[21-23], systematic review[24] and integration of available data on a given problem as originally presented in psychology and education. Medicine has adopted, adapted and further developed this search for evidence.

In medicine, we have defined meta-analysis as ' . . . *a systematic, organized and structured evaluation and synthesis of a problem of interest based on results of many independent studies of that problem (disease cause, treatment effect, diagnostic method, prognosis, etc.)*[21,10] . . .'. In such an 'epidemiological study of studies' results', the quality of studies is assessed first (qualitative meta-analysis) and then numerical results are integrated statistically (quantitative meta-analysis) to determine if treatment works or if an agent is harmful to health.

In EBM, the best evidence is combined with other components of clinical decision making[25,26]. It should include individual clinical expertise, knowledge from basic sciences, and patient preferences and values. Presently, many questions related to this process remain only partially answered[27]. What clinical knowledge and experience is relevant? Which criteria allow experience and evidence to be combined? Which criteria favour experience over evidence or vice versa? How should experience and evidence be weighed? Are there any flow charts that organize in time and space the steps required to combine evidence and experience?

If establishing the nature of 'best evidence' is problematic, is it actually possible for us to properly grasp the concept of evidence-based medicine itself? Does the best evidence work as a 'filter' in medicine in terms of Figure 2.1?

2.4 WHAT IS EVIDENCE-BASED MEDICINE?

EBM brings organization and structure to medical decisions just as decision analysis or cost-effectiveness analysis already do, but in a different way. Table 2.1 summarizes two common definitions of EBM and shows how the concept fully applies to **evidence-based public health** (EBPH)[27]. It also indicates the steps required for both of these practices.

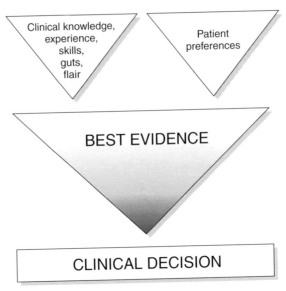

Figure 2.1 – Filter of best evidence. Source: Reference 27

EBM with its emphasis on evidence is the opposite of fringe medicines, alternative medicines, or complementary medicines, grouped by Cocker[28] into the category of **'claims-based medicine'**, i.e. *'. . . that's how it is because I'm telling you that that's how it is! . . . Evidence? Come on! It's obvious! . . . '*

One of the logical outgrowths of the EBM concept is **evidence-based health care**, i.e. *'. . . a discipline centred upon evidence-based decision making about individual patients, groups of patients or populations, which may be manifest as evidence-based purchasing or evidence-based management.'*[29]

For health care decisions, Stevens[30] proposes more than an evidence-based approach through **knowledge-based health service**: *' . . . health care decisions (whether about a patient or a population) need to be focused on research-based evidence about the consequences of treatment **augmented** by the intelligent use of wider information on, for example, finance, patient flows and healthcare politics . . . '*

EBM must be seen as a permanently evolving process in order to keep up with the pace of rapidly evolving experience and research production in health sciences. As an example, Aspirin® may at first be considered the analgesic and/or antipyretic of choice for some patients. However, at a later time, because of

Table 2.1 – Definition and steps of evidence-based medicine and evidence-based public health Source: References 25, 26 and 27

Evidence-based medicine (EBM)	Evidence-based public health (EBPH)
Definition The process of systematically finding, appraising, and using contemporaneous research findings as the basis for clinical decisions *or:* The conscientious, explicit, and judicious use of current best evidence in making decisions about the care of individual patients	**Definition** The process of systematically finding, appraising, and using contemporaneous clinical and community research findings as the basis for decisions in public health *or:* The conscientious, explicit, and judicious use of current best evidence in making decisions about the care of communities and populations in the domain of health protection, disease prevention, and health maintenance and improvement (health promotion)
Steps of its practice ● Formulation of a clear question from a patient's problem which has to be answered ● Searching the literature for relevant articles and exploring other sources of information ● Critical appraisal of the evidence (information provided by original research or by research synthesis, i.e. systematic reviews and meta-analysis) ● Selection of the best evidence or useful findings for clinical decision ● Linking evidence with clinical experience, knowledge, and practice and with the patient's values and preferences ● Implementation of useful findings in clinical practice ● Evaluation of the implementation and overall performance of the EBM practitioner, and ● Teaching others how to practise EBM	**Steps of its practice** ● Formulation of a clear question arising from a public health problem ● Searching for evidence ● Appraisal of evidence ● Selection of the best evidence for a public health decision ● Linking evidence with public health experience, knowledge, and practice and with the community values and preferences ● Implementation of useful evidences in public health practice (policies and programs) ● Evaluation of such implementations and of the overall performance of the EBPH practitioner, and ● Teaching others how to practise EBPH
*Its goal: **The best possible management of health and disease in individual patient(s).***	*Its goal: **The best possible management of health and disease and their determinants at the community level***

Aspirin's® adverse effects, the patients may be given Tylenol® instead.

EBM is approximately one decade 'young'. Since its inception[1], EBM has been the subject of an ongoing series of articles in the *Journal of the American Medical Association* (*JAMA*)[29-54]. EBM theory and practice appear in a 'little red book'[55](now a 'little blue book'[56]) and other valuable monographs[57-59]. The search for evidence has also been outlined[60] and short introductory articles[61-63] have focused on it as well. Even related training programs have been created[64].

Several new journals have been launched such as *Evidence Based Medicine*, the *ACP Journal Club* (American College of Physicians' Journal Club), *Evidence-Based Nursing*, and *Evidence-Based Mental Health*. French-speaking readers have access to *EBM Journal. Evidence-Based-Medicine. Relier la Recherche aux Pratiques. Édition française (Un journal de l'American College of Physicians et du BMJ Publishing Group)*.

The evidence-based approach has also expanded and been applied to other specialties and fields, such as:

- Community medicine and health care[29, 65-69]
- Public health[27, 70-77]
- Health promotion[78]
- Surgery[79-80]
- Emergency medicine[81,82]
- Inpatient medicine[83], general practice[84], family practice[85,86], primary care[87,88]
- Mental health services[89] and psychiatry[90]
- Psychosomatic medicine[91]
- Obstetrics and gynaecology[92]
- Neurology[93]
- Nephrology[94-97]
- Clinical biochemistry[98]
- Diagnostic radiology[99]
- Coronary care[100]
- Paediatrics[101-103]
- Otolaryngology[104]
- Geriatric medicine[105]
- Hepatology[106]

- Audiology[107]
- Laboratory medicine[108]
- Cancer care[109]
- Anaesthesiology[110,111]
- Hospital epidemiology (infection control)[112]
- Gastroenterology[113]
- Internal medicine[114]
- Sport sciences and medicine[115]
- Ophthalmology[116]

and other health sciences beyond the above mentioned medical domains, like dentistry[117–120], nursing[121–123] and acupuncture[124].

Views and opinions about EBM are still not unanimous. For example, the same introductory article[117] about EBM has elicited the following Letters to the Editor:

> 'The article... could be the most important relevant scientific article I have ever read in my life...'[25]

but also

> '. . . Quite frankly, this is the most specious and useless piece of garbage that I have encountered since I graduated from dental school.'[126]

As it happens often, the truth is somewhere in between as we may see it across the literature and lived experience.

The growing acceptance of EBM as a novel way of reasoning and decision making in medicine is inevitably accompanied by **critiques and calls for caution**, already reviewed elsewhere[27] and still being produced[20, 80, 127–142]. In essence, these critiques call for a non-dogmatic use of EBM as a replacement for everything else in medicine and its link and integration with the 'old arts'[127,86] of medicine, basic sciences, patient or social (community) values[140].

In reality, EBM should take into account clinical spectrum, gradient, clinimetric stratification and prognostic characteristics of disease[20].

Recommendations and guidelines may be made only when individual characteristics are compatible with those in the research and synthesis. Linking 'group evidence'[82] and the value of evidence for a specific patient[85] remains a great challenge[85,86]. EBM's application to the individual patient remains a cornerstone of its further development.

Randomized controlled trials, considered among the best source of evidence of cause–effect relationships, cannot answer all clinical questions in medicine. For ethical and technical reasons[129,134], these studies are not always feasible.

The scope of EBM is larger than EB treatment. Qualitative research[143,144], observational, descriptive and analytical studies[145,146], diagnosis[147,148], screening[149–151], prognosis, or ethics[152–154] pose additional challenges in terms of relevance and justified use in EBM. These fields as well as treatment effectiveness research should be further developed and physicians should be properly trained in all these practices[155–157].

Why is EBM so challenging? We can agree with Kernick[132] that ' ... *decisions in life are based on a cognitive continuum. Wired to the cardiological bed, the heart disease succumbs to inferential statistics. But patients come and go: to the real world where attempts to impose a spurious rationality on an irrational process may not always succeed; where structures are highly complex and disease thresholds may not be met; where decisions are based on past experience, future expectations, and complex human inter-relationships; where doctors and patients have their own narratives* (and their own values and priorities!); *where time scales exceed those of the longest trial; and where the mechanisms of poverty are the greatest of dysease ...'.* Barriers overcome and bridges built[158], EBM remains a relevant and rewarding experience for patients, their physicians and their health planners and managers.

The philosophy and emerging practice of EBM as well as its related clinical case reporting, may be summarized as follows:

- 'Evidence' is based on real-life observations.
- 'Evidence' is not a decision itself; however, good evidence is needed to make good decisions.
- The evolution from practice and 'soft' experience

to evidence-based experience has not yet been universally achieved.

- More evidence does not necessarily mean more EBM practice.
- Clinical research means *systematic* clinical observations.
- Clinical research evolves from an unsystematic gathering, analysis, interpretation, and use of data and information to a systematic and *integrated approach*.
- EBM is primarily about thinking. Computing and use of information technology are strictly considered supportive tools.
- EBM reflects a deterministic/probabilistic shift in today's paradigm of medicine dealing with uncertainty. EBM is more evolutionary than revolutionary.
- With EBM, clinical epidemiology is within the reach of all health professionals in today's information-based world.
- Changes in thinking, not textbooks, affect the way medicine is practised.
- More cases where EBM is used are necessary. A number of *ad hoc* seminars are not sufficient.
- EBM lends itself perfectly to problem and/or system-oriented teaching.
- EBM mastery does not replace clinical skills and experience. It organizes, expands and completes them.
- Just as Flexnerian* reform transformed medicine from erratic usage of experience and educated guesses to its modern scientific basis in North America, the EBM movement is considered another contemporary change in the way medicine is practised.

---

* Abraham Flexner (1910), a physician who wrote a report which opened the way to the radical improvement of teaching and practice of medicine in North America.

- There must be an important trade-off between administrative, authoritative and authoritarian decisions on the one hand, and quality evidence-based judgements and their applications on the other.

As for **clinical case applications**:

- In case-based situations, there will be an increasing number of links between pattern recognition and a systematic evidence-based approach.
- The 'underdog' status of working with clinical cases must be overcome, as it has already been done in more conclusive research based on single or multiple case observations.

Some **contrasts in the EBM concept** (i.e. 'one thing does not mean another') must be kept in mind:

- Use of computers and databases vs. the way these tools are worked with, and the way conclusions are drawn about problems.
- Instinct and thinking vs. working with evidence and making decisions based on the best evidence available.
- 'Primary' studies on risk, diagnosis, treatment, prognosis, or decisions vs. 'integrative' studies with systematic reviews, clinical guidelines, algorithms and other clinician guides focusing on the most efficient, effective, and efficacious preventions and cures in the whole care and management of individual patients and groups of individuals.

2.5 WHAT DOES THE FUTURE HOLD FOR EBM?

EBM is a topic that many luminaries love to hate. Nevertheless, EBM is here to stay, because there will always be a need to find the elusive 'best evidence' in medicine.

And the future of EBM?

- It should not become a 'cookbook medicine'[159].
- It will rely on an increasingly complex surveillance of evidence like that performed by the Cochrane Collaboration[160].
- In order to succeed, it will have to integrate elements from various fields of medicine and public health (see Figure 2.2)[27].
- It will overcome the challenge of applying the best evidence to individual patients while making them an integral part of decision making[161–163].
- EBM decisions will be increasingly accountable in courts of law[164,165].
- It will be increasingly considered a competency[166].
- Its success should be evaluable and evaluated[167].
- It should be 'sold' as 'medicine with a human face' despite its important technically sophisticated components, such as information retrieval and research synthesis (meta-analysis). Thus, it will make a place for itself somewhere between bedside clinical work with the patient and decision analysis and making[169] (see Figure 2.3).
- It will be increasingly used by health policy makers[167].

The future of EBM is clouded by the reality of the present state of medicine[170] which, at the same time, is its *raison d'être*. Some causes of this situation[170] are worthy of attention:

- Actions which do not always take into account scientific advancements.

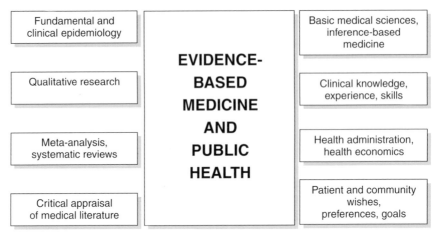

Fundamental and clinical epidemiology		Basic medical sciences, inference-based medicine
Qualitative research	**EVIDENCE-BASED MEDICINE AND PUBLIC HEALTH**	Clinical knowledge, experience, skills
Meta-analysis, systematic reviews		Health administration, health economics
Critical appraisal of medical literature		Patient and community wishes, preferences, goals

Figure 2.2 – Evidence-based medicine and evidence-based public health: an ambitious integration? Source: Reference 27

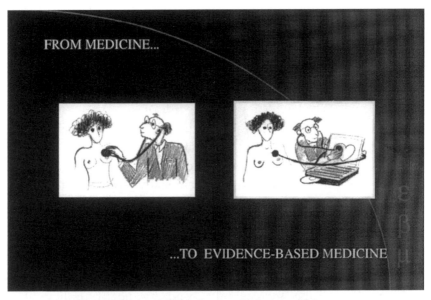

Figure 2.3 – The challenge of EBM. Source: Reference 168

- Lack of consistency and objectivity of observers.
- Frequent omission of crucial clinical details in evidence building and decision making.
- Authoritarianism of 'authorities'.
- Excessive generalizations from research and experience on phenomena with limited clinical spectrum, gradient, and prognosis.

2.6 DO CLINICAL CASE REPORTS PLAY A ROLE IN THE PRESENT AND FUTURE OF EBM?

In answer to the above question, clinical case reports definitely play a role in the present and future of EBM.

However, as relatively modest as evidence case reports might be, they remain a frequent source of evidence. In fact, several specialties including clinical microbiology, psychiatry and surgery rely heavily on case reports as evidence. Figure 2.4 shows how important case reports and case series reports were in the core paediatric surgery literature[171] during the period from 1996 to 1997. This is the starting point for clinical experience and more advanced research.

In terms of EBM, a clinical case report can be viewed from two different angles:

- It is a source of evidence, and
- An evidence-based approach and evidence itself are needed in the interpretation of the case and in its clinical management.

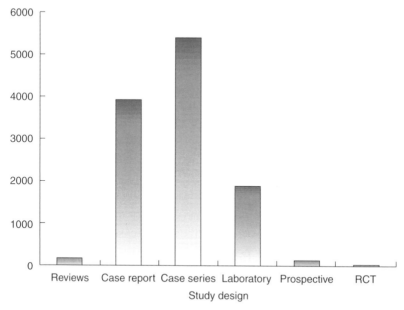

Figure 2.4 – Dominance of case reports and case series reports. An example from the core paediatric surgery literature 1966–1997. Source: Reference 171

The first angle leads to the development of an '**evidence-based case report**'. As an example, in a case of an induced labour, subsequent uterine rupture and fetal death at delivery, Vause and Macintosh[172] overviewed evidence related to the use of prostaglandins and oxytocin while awaiting or inducing labour in women with previous caesarean section. Evidence was gathered from randomized controlled trials, non-randomized cohort studies and case–control studies. There was insufficient evidence to support the **development of a 'beyond the case guideline'** on whether women with previous caesarean section scar should or should not be offered induction with prostaglandins. However, the fringe benefit of this case experience was openness to the introduction of an evidence-based medicine approach in the clinical department.

With respect to the second angle, Browman[173] shows how available evidence can and should be used in an individual case of prostate cancer. A treatment with biophosphonates and hormonal/radiotherapy option was discussed with an intelligent patient on the basis of available evidence and the patient's preferences. **An evidence-based individualized solution was therefore sought in this particular case**. A reasonable clinical decision was made by the patient in a situation of indirect evidence of benefit that would be insufficient to support the same decision as a health policy beyond the case.

Case reports, however, can go well beyond individual patient experience. Vandenbroucke[174,175] rightly points out that case reports can contribute to descriptions of new diseases and develop the first ideas about aetiology and recognition of side effects, about disease mechanisms, therapy and prognosis. They contribute to the quality assurance of clinical care, i.e. suggesting 'what to do in order to not make the same mistake'. As a teaching tool, they show young clinicians how to think.

In many specialized fields of medicine (i.e. surgery, clinical microbiology, toxicology, psychiatry, genetics, traumatology, emergency medicine, or occupational medicine), cases are rare and clinical trials cannot always be performed for technical, economical, and/or ethical reasons. Thus, case reports become an important part of evidence.

As for the use of evidence in decision making in a specific clinical case, more experience from a wider use of evidence-based case management is needed at this point in the development of evidence-based medicine and clinical case management and reporting.

A clinical case report can be seen in Enkin and Jadad's terms[176] as an 'anecdote', i.e. a brief account of some incident; a short narrative of an interesting or entertaining nature[13]. However, this does not mean that a clinical case report is necessarily anecdotal! Even serious accounts, which complement even more serious endeavours, require their own set of rules, as outlined on the following pages.

REFERENCES

1. Evidence-Based Medicine Working Group (G Guyatt *et al.*). Evidence-based medicine. A new approach to teaching practice of medicine. *JAMA*, 1992; **268**: 2420–5.
2. Morris JN. *Uses of Epidemiology*. Edinburgh and London: Livingstone, 1967.
3. MacMahon B, Pugh TF. *Epidemiology. Principles and Methods*. Boston: Little, Brown, 1970.
4. Roberts CJ. *Epidemiology for Clinicians*. Tunbridge Wells: Pitman Medical, 1977.
5. Fletcher RH, Fletcher SW, Wagner EH. *Clinical Epidemiology – the Essentials*. Baltimore: Williams & Wilkins, 1982.
6. Sackett DL, Haynes RB, Tugwell PX. *Clinical Epidemiology. A Basic Science for Clinical Practice*. Boston: Little, Brown, 1984.
7. Feinstein AR. *Clinical Epidemiology. The Architecture of Clinical Research*. Philadelphia: WB Saunders, 1985.
8. Jenicek M, Cléroux R. *Épidémiologie clinique. Clinimétrie (Clinical Epidemiology. Clinimetrics.)* St Hyacinthe and Paris: EDISEM and Maloine, 1985.
9. *A Dictionary of Epidemiology*, Third Edition. Edited by JM Last. New York, Oxford, Toronto: Oxford University Press, 1995.
10. Jenicek M. *Epidemiology. The Logic of Modern Medicine*. Montreal: EPIMED International, 1995.
11. Feinstein AR. An additional science for clinical medicine: IV. The development of clinimetrics. *Ann Intern Med*, 1983; **99**: 843–8.
12. Feinstein AR. *Clinimetrics*. New Haven: Yale University Press, 1987.
13. *New Illustrated Webster's Dictionary of the English Language*. New York: PAMCO Publishing Company, 1992.
14. Auclair F. On the nature of evidence. *Annals RCPSC*, 1999; **32**: 453–5.
15. Loomis D, Wing S. Is molecular epidemiology a germ theory for the end of the twentieth century? *Int J Epidemiol*,1990; **19**: 1–3.
16. Perera FP, Weinstein BI. Molecular epidemiology and carcinogen-DNA adduct detection: New approaches to studies of human cancer causation. *J Chronic Dis*, 1982; **35**: 581–600.

17. Schull WJ, Weiss KM. Genetic epidemiology : four strategies. *Epidemiol Rev*, 1980; **2**: 1–18.

18. The Canadian Task Force on the Periodic Health Examination. *The Canadian Guide to Clinical Preventive Health Care*. Ottawa: Health Canada, 1994.

19. Sackett DL. Rules of evidence and clinical recommendations. *Can J Cardiol*, 1993; **9**: 487–9.

20. Feinstein AR, Horwitz RI. Problems in the 'evidence' of 'evidence-based medicine'. *Am J Med*, 1997; **103**: 529–35.

21. Jenicek M. Meta-analysis in medicine. Where we are and where we want to go. *J Clin Epidemiol*, 1989; **42**: 35–44.

22. Petitti DB. *Meta-analysis, Decision Analysis, and Cost-Effectiveness Analysis. Methods of Quantitative Synthesis in Medicine*. Monographs in Epidemiology and Biostatistics, Volume 24. New York and Oxford: Oxford University Press, 1994.

23. Jenicek M. *Méta-analyse en médecine. Evaluation et synthèse de l'information clinique et épidémiologique. (Meta-analysis in Medicine. Evaluation and Synthesis of Clinical and Epidemiological Information.)* St Hyacinthe and Paris: EDISEM and Maloine, 1987.

24. Cook DJ, Mulrow CD, Haynes RB. Systematic reviews: Synthesis of best evidence for clinical decisions. *Ann Intern Med*, 1997; **126**: 376–80.

25. Rosenberg W, Donald A. Evidence based medicine: an approach to clinical problem-solving. *BMJ*, 1995; **310**: 1122–6.

26. Sackett DL, Rosenberg WMC, Muir Gray JA, Haynes RB, Richardson WS. Evidence-based medicine: what it is and what it isn't. *BMJ*, 1996; **312**: 71–2.

27. Jenicek M. Epidemiology, evidence-based medicine, and evidence-based public health. *J Epidemiol*, 1997; **7**: 187–97.

28. Cocker J. Henry VIII and I. *Stitches*, 1999, No. 92: 76–8.

29. Muir Gray JA. *Evidence-based healthcare. How to Make Health Policy and Management Decisions*. New York: Churchill Livingstone, 1997.

30. Stevens A. A knowledge-based health service: how do the new initiatives work? *J Roy Soc Med*, 1998; **91**(Suppl. No. 35): 26–31.

31. Oxman AD, Sackett DL, Guyatt GH for the Evidence-Based Medicine Working Group. User's guides to the medical literature. I. How to get started. *JAMA*, 1993; **270**: 2093–5.

32. Guyatt GH, Sackett DL, Cook DJ for the Evidence-Based Medicine Working Group. User's guides to the medical literature. II. How to use an article about therapy or prevention. A. Are the results valid? *JAMA*, 1993; **270**: 2598–601. B. What were the results and will they help me in caring for my patients? *JAMA*, 1994; **271**: 59–63.

33. Jaeschke R, Guyatt G, Sackett DL for the Evidence-Based Medicine Working Group. Users' guides to the medical literature. III. How to use an article about a diagnostic test. A. Are the results of the study valid? *JAMA*, 1994; **271**: 389–91. B. What are the results and will they help me in caring for my patients? Idem: 703–7.

34. Levine M, Walter S, Lee H, Haines T, Holbrook A, Moyer V for the Evidence-

Based Medicine Working Group. Users' guides to the medical literature. IV. How to use an article about harm. *JAMA*, 1994; **271**: 1615–9.

35. Laupacis A, Wells G, Richardson S, Tugwell P for the Evidence-Based Medicine Working Group. Users' guides to the medical literature. V. How to use an article about prognosis. *JAMA*, 1994; **272**: 234–7.

36. Oxman AD, Cook DJ, Guyatt GH for the Evidence-Based Medicine Working Group. Users' guides to the medical literature. VI. How to use an overview. *JAMA*, 1994; **272**: 1367–71.

37. Richardson SW, Detsky AS for the Evidence-Based Medicine Working Group. Users' guides to the medical literature. VII. How to use a clinical decision analysis. A. Are the results of the study valid? *JAMA*, 1995; **273**: 1292–5. B. What are the results and will they help me in caring for my patients? *JAMA*, 1995; **273**: 1610–3.

38. Hayward RSA, Wilson MC, Tunis SR, Bass EB, Guyatt G for the Evidence-Based Medicine Working Group. Users' guides to the medical literature. VIII. How to use clinical practice guidelines. A. Are the recommendations valid? *JAMA*, 1995; **274**: 570–4.

39. Wilson MC, Hayward SA, Tunis SR, Bass EB, Guyatt G for the Evidence-Based Medicine Working Group. Users' guides to the medical literature. VIII. How to use clinical practice guidelines. B. What are the recommendations and will they help you in caring for your patients? *JAMA*, 1995; **274**: 1630–2.

40. Guyatt GH, Sackett DL, Sinclair JC, Hayward R, Cook DJ, Cook RJ for the Evidence-Based Medicine Working Group. Users' guides to the medical literature. IX. A method for grading health care recommendations. *JAMA*, 1995; **274**: 1800–4.

41. Naylor CD, Guyatt GH for the Evidence-Based Medicine Working Group. Users' guides to the medical literature. X. How to use an article reporting variations in the outcomes of health services. *JAMA*, 1996; **275**: 554–8.

42. Naylor CD, Guyatt GH for the Evidence-Based Medicine Working Group. Users' guides to the medical literature. XI. How to use an article about a clinical utilization review. *JAMA*, 1996; **275**: 1435–9.

43. Guyatt GH, Naylor CD, Juniper E, Heyland DK, Jaeschke R, Cook DJ for the Evidence-Based Medicine Working Group. Users' guides to the medical literature. XII. How to use articles about health-related quality of life. *JAMA*, 1997; **277**: 1232–7.

44. Drummond MF, Richardson SW, O'Brien BJ, Levine M, Heyland D for the Evidence-Based Medicine Working Group. Users' guides to the medical literature. XIII. How to use an article on economic analysis of clinical practice. A. Are the results of the study valid? *JAMA*, 1997; **277**: 1552–7.

45. O'Brien BJ, Heyland D, Richardson WS, Levine M, Drummond MF for the Evidence-Based Medicine Working Group. Users' guides to the medical literature. XIII. B. What are the results and will they help me in caring for my patients? *JAMA*, 1997; **277**: 1802–6.

46. Dans AL, Dans LF, Guyatt GH, Richardson S for the Evidence-Based Medicine Working Group. Users' guides to the medical literature. XIV. How to decide

on the applicability of clinical trial results to your patient. *JAMA*, 1998; **279**: 545–9.

47. Richardson WS, Wilson MC, Guyatt GH, Cook DJ, Nishikawa J for the Evidence-Based Medicine Working Group. Users' guides to the medical literature. XV. How to use an article about disease probability for differential diagnosis. *JAMA*, 199; **281**: 1214–9.

48. Guyatt GH, Sinclair J, Cook DJ, Glasziou P for the Evidence-Based Medicine Working Group and the Cochrane Applicability Methods Working Group. Users' guides to the medical literature. XVI. How to use a treatment recommendation. *JAMA*, 1999; **281**: 1836–43.

49. Barratt A, Irwig L, Glasziou P, Cumming RG, Raffle A, Hicks N, Muir Gray JA, Guyatt GH for the Evidence-Based Medicine Working Group. Users' guides to the medical literature. XVII. How to use guidelines and recommendations about screening. *JAMA*, 1999; **281**: 2029–34.

50. Randolph AG, Haynes RB, Wyatt JC, Cook DJ, Guyatt GH. Users' guides to the medical literature. XVIII. How to use an article evaluating the clinical impact of a computer-based clinical decision support system. *JAMA*, 1999; **282**: 67–74.

51. Bucher HC, Guyatt GH, Cook DJ, Holbrook A, McAlister FA for the Evidence-Based Medicine Working Group. XIX. Applying clinical trial results. A. How to use an article measuring the effect of an intervention on surrogate end points. *JAMA*, 1999; **282**: 771–8.

52. McAlister FA, Laupacis A, Wells GA, Sackett DL for the Evidence-Based Medicine Working Group. Users' guides to the medical literature. XIX. Applying clinical trial results. B. Guidelines for determining whether a drug is exerting (more than) a class effect. *JAMA*, 1999; **282**: 1371–7.

53. McAlister FA, Straus SE, Guyatt GH, Haynes RB for the Evidence-Based Medicine Working Group. Users' guides to the medical literature. XX. Integrating research evidence with the care of the individual patient. *JAMA*, 2000; **283**: 2829–36.

54. Hunt DL, Jaeschke R, McKibbon KA for the Evidence-Based Medicine Working Group. Users' guides to the medical literature. XXI. Using electronic health information resources in evidence-based practice. *JAMA*, 2000; **283**: 1875–9.

55. Sackett DL, Richardson WS, Rosenberg W, Haynes RB. *Evidence-Based Medicine. How to Practice and Teach EBM*. New York: Churchill Livingstone, 1997.

56. Sackett DL, Straus SE, Richardson SW, Rosenberg W, Haynes RB. *Evidence-Based Medicine. How to Practice and Teach EBM*, 2nd Edition. Edinburgh and London: Churchill Livingstone, 2000.

57. Dixon RA, Munro JF, Silcocks PB. *The Evidence Based Medicine Workbook. Critical Appraisal for Clinical Problem Solving*. Oxford: Butterworth Heinemann, 1997.

58. *Evidence-Based Practice*. Edited by M Daves *et al*. Edinburgh: Churchill Livingstone, 1999.

59. *Achieving Evidence Based Practice.* Edited by S Hamer and G Collinson. Edinburgh: Baillière Tindall, 1999.

60. McKibbon KA, Marks S, Eady A. *PDQ Evidence-Based Principles and Practice.* Hamilton: BC Decker Inc., 1999.

61. Bigby M. Evidence-based medicine in a nutshell. A guide to finding and using the best evidence in caring for patients. *Arch Dermatol,* 1998; **134**: 1609–18.

62. Etminan M, Wright JM, Carleton BC. Evidence-based pharmacotherapy: review of basic concepts and applications in clinical practice. *Ann Pharmacother,* 1998; **32**: 1193–200.

63. Green L. Using evidence-based medicine in clinical practice. *Oncology,* 1998; **25**: 391–400.

64. Greenhalgh T, Donald A. *Evidence Based Health Care Workbook: understanding research. For individual and group learning.* London: BMJ Books, 2000.

65. Evidence-Based Care Resource Group (Oxman AD, principal coauthor). Evidence-based care: 1. Setting priorities: How important is the problem? *CMAJ,* 1994; **150**: 1249–54. 2. Setting guidelines: How should we manage the problem? Idem: 1417–23. 3. Measuring performance: How are we managing this problem? Idem: 1575–9. 4. Improving performance: How can we improve the way we manage this problem? Idem: 1793–6. 5. Lifelong learning: How can we learn to be more effective? Idem: 1971–3.

66. Reerink E, Walshe K. Evidence-based healthcare: a critical appraisal. *J Roy Soc Med,*1998 (Suppl. No. 35); **91**: 1.

67. Firth-Cozens J. Healthy promotion: changing behaviour towards evidence-based health care. *Qual Health Care,* 1997; **6**(4): 205–11.

68. Michaud G, McGowan JL, van der Jagt R, Wells G, Tugwell P. Are therapeutic decisions supported by evidence from health care research? *Arch Intern Med,* 1998; **158**: 1665–8.

69. Chalfin DB. Evidence-based medicine and cost-effectiveness analysis. *Crit Care Clinics,* 1998; **1**(No. 3): 525–37.

70. Lohr KN, Eleazer K, Mauskopf J. Health policy issues and applications for evidence-based medicine and clinical practice guidelines. *Health Policy,* 1998; **46**: 1–19.

71. Frater A. Quality of care in developing countries: relevance and reality. *Qual Health Care,* 1997; **6**: 179–80.

72. Harries U, Elliott H, Higgins A. Evidence-based policy-making in the NHS: exploring the interface between research and the commissioning process. *J Public Health Med,* 1999; **21**: 29–36.

73. Dickersin K, Manheimer E. The Cochrane Collaboration: evaluation of health care and services using systematic reviews of the results of randomized clinical trials. *Clin Obstet Gynecol,* 1998; **41**: 15–31.

74. Aveyard P. Evidence-based medicine and public health. *J Eval Clin Pract,* 1997; **3**: 139–44.

75. Wagner M. The public health versus clinical approaches to maternity services: the emperor has no clothes. *J Public Health Policy,* 1998; **19**: 25–35.

76. Glasziou P, Longbottom H. Evidence-based public health practice. *Aust NZ J Public Health*, 1999; **23**: 436–40.
77. Brownson RC *et al*. Evidence-based decision making in public health. *J Public Health Manag Pract*, 1999; **5**: 86–97.
78. *Evidence-based Health Promotion*. Edited by ER Perkins, I Simnett, L Wright. Chichester and New York: J Wiley, 1999.
79. Black N. Evidence-based surgery: A passing fad? *World J Surg*, 1999; **23**: 789–93.
80. Evidence-Based Surgery. Edited by TA Gordon and JL Cameron. Hamilton and London: BC Decker Inc., 2000.
81. Guyatt GH. Evidence-based emergency medicine. *Ann Emerg Med*, 1997; **30**: 675–6.
82. Waeckerle JF, Cordell WH, Wyer P, Osborn HH. Evidence-based emergency medicine: Integrating research into practice. *Ann Emerg Med*, 1997; **30**: 626–8.
83. Ellis J, Mulligan I, Towe J, Sackett DL. On behalf of the A-team, Nuffield Department of Clinical Medicine. Inpatient general medicine is evidence based. *Lancet*, 1995; **346**: 407–10.
84. Jacobson LD, Edwards AGK, Granier SK, Butler CC. Evidence-based medicine and general practice. *Br J Gen Pract*, 1997; **47**: 449–52.
85. MacAuley D. The integration of evidence based medicine and personal care in family practice. *Irish J Med Sci*, 1996; **165**: 289–91.
86. Rosser WW, Shafir MS. *Evidence-Based Family Medicine*. Hamilton and London: BC Decker, 1998.
87. Geyman JP. Evidence-based medicine in primary care: an overview. *J Am Board Fam Pract*, 1998; **11**: 46–56.
88. *Evidence-Based Clinical Practice: Concepts and Approaches*. Edited by JP Geyman, RA Deyo, SD Ramsey. Boston and Oxford: Butterworth Heinemann, 2000.
89. Barnes J, Stein A, Rosenberg W. Evidence based medicine and evaluation of mental health services: methodological issues and future directions. *Arch Dis Child*, 1999; **80**: 280–5.
90. Goldner EM, Bilsker D. Evidence-based psychiatry, *Can J Psychiatry*, 1995; **40**: 97–101.
91. Sharpe M, Gill D, Strain J, Mayou R. Psychosomatic medicine and evidence-based treatment. *J Psychosom Res*, 1996; **41**: 101–7.
92. Grimes DA. Introducing evidence-based medicine into a department of obstetrics and gynecology. *Obstet Gynecol*, 1995; **86**: 451–7. Correspondence: Idem, 1996; **87**: 169–160.
93. Longstreth WT Jr., Psaty BM. When you look for evidence and find too much. *Neurology*, 1998; **50**: 544–6.
94. Fouque D, Laville M, Haugh M, Boissel JP. Systematic reviews and their role in promoting evidence-based medicine in renal disease. *Nephrol Dial Transplant*, 1996; **11**: 2398–401.
95. Haugh M, Fouque D. Evidence-based nephrology. *Neurol Dial Transplant*, 1999; **14**(Suppl. 3): 38–41.
96. Zoccali C. Evidence-based medicine: the clinician's perspective. *Neurol Dial Transplant*, 1999; **14**(Suppl. 3): 42–5.

97. Liberati A, Telaro E, Perna A. Evidence-based medicine and its horizons: a useful tool for nephrologists? *Nephrol Dial Transplant*, 1999; **14**(Suppl. 3): 46–52.

98. Moore RA. Evidence-based clinical biochemistry. *Ann Clin Biochem*, 1997; **34**: 3–7.

99. Dixon AK. Evidence-based diagnostic radiology. *Lancet*, 1997; **350**: 509–12.

100. Braunwald E, Antman EM. Evidence-based coronary care. *Ann Intern Med*, 1997; **126**: 551–3.

101. Gilbert R, Logan S. Future prospects for evidence-based child health. *Arch Dis Childhood*, 1996; **75**: 465–73.

102. Elliott EJ, Moyer VA. Evidence-based pediatrics. *J Pediat Child Health*, 1998; **34**: 14–7.

103. *Evidence-Based Pediatrics.* Edited by W Feldman. Hamilton: BC Decker, 2000.

104. Gibbin KP. Evidence based medicine in otolaryngology. *J Laryngol Otol*, 1997; **111**: 415–7.

105. Burns R, Pahor M, Shorr RI. Evidence-based medicine holds the key to the future for geriatric medicine. *JAGS (J Am Geriatr Soc)*, 1997; **45**: 1268–72.

106. Younossi Z, Guyatt G. Evidence-based medicine: A method for solving clinical problems in hepatology. *Hepatology*, 1999; **30**: 829–32.

107. Robinson K. Evidence-based medicine and its implications for audiological science. *Br J Audiol*, 1999; **33**: 9–16.

108. Moore RA. Concepts and principles of evidence-based laboratory medicine. *Am Clin Lab*, 1999; **18**: 24–5.

109. Williams CJ. Evidence-based cancer care. *Clin Oncol (R Coll Radiol)*, 1998; **10**: 144–9.

110. Horan BF. Evidence-based medicine and anaesthesia: uneasy bedfellows? *Anaesth Intensive Care*, 1997; **25**: 679–85.

111. Tramèr MR. What can systematic reviews teach us in anaesthesia? *Acta Anaesthesiol Scand,* Suppl., 1997; **111**: 235–6.

112. Jenner EA *et al.* Infection control – evidence into practice. *J Hosp Infect*, 1999; **42**: 91–104.

113. Schoenfeld P, Cook D, Hamilton F, Laine L, Morgan D, Peterson W. An evidence-based approach to gastroenterology therapy. Evidence-Based Gastroenterology Steering Group. *Gastroenterology*, 1998; **114**: 1318–25.

114. *Quick Consult Manual of Evidence-Based Medicine.* Edited by BW Lee, SI Hsu, DS Stasior. Philadelphia and New York: Lippincott–Raven Publishers, 1997.

115. Biddle S. Chaos in the brickyard revisited: in research integration, accumulated knowledge and evidence-based practice in the exercise and sport sciences. *J Sport Sci*, 1997; **15**: 383–4.

116. Sharma S. Levels of evidence and interventional ophthalmology. *Can J Ophthalmol*, 1997; **32**: 356–62.

117. Raphael K, Marbach JJ. Evidence-based care of musculoskeletal facial pain: implications for the clinical science of dentistry. *JADA*, 1997; **128**: 73–7.

118. Newman MG. Improved clinical decision making using the evidence-based approach. *Ann Periodontol*, 1996 (Nov); **1**: i–ix.

119. Dodson TB. Evidence-based medicine. Its role in the modern practice and teaching of dentistry. *Oral Surg Oral Med Oral Pathol Oral Radiol Endod*, 1997; **83**: 192–7.

120. Nainar SM. Evidence-based dental care – a concept review. *Pediatr Dent*, 1998; **20**: 418–21.

121. Simpson B. Evidence-based nursing practice. The state of the art. *Can Nurse*, 1996(Nov); **92**: 22–5.

122. Shorten A, Wallace M. Evidence-based practice. The future is clear. *Austr Nurs J*, 1996(Dec 1996–Jan 1997); **4**: 22–4.

123. Gagliardi A. Ontario Health Care Evaluation Network: Building partnership and promoting evidence-based practice. *Can J Nurs Res*, 1996; **28**: 145–9.

124. Ullet GA *et al.* Traditional and evidence-based acupuncture: history, mechanisms, and present status. *South Med J*, 1998; **91**: 1115–20.

125. Niamtu J, III. Evidence-based care. Letter to The Editor. *JADA*, 1997; **128**: 402–3.

126. Cook TR III. A contrasting view. Letter to The Editor. *JADA*, 1997; **128**: 403.

127. Naylor CD. Grey zones of clinical practice: some limits to evidence-based medicine. *Lancet*, 1995; **345**: 840–2.

128. Cohn JN. Evidence-based medicine: What is the evidence? *J Cardiac Failure*, 1996; **2**: 159–161.

129. Polychronis A, Miles AS, Bentley P. Evidence-based medicine: reference? Dogma? Neologism? New Orthodoxy? *J Eval Clin Pract*, 1996; **2**: 1–3.

130. Polychronis A, Miles A, Bentley P. The protagonists of 'evidence-based medicine': arrogant, seductive and controversial. *J Eval Clin Pract*, 1996; **2**: 9–12.

131. Kenny NP. Does good science make good medicine? Incorporating evidence into practice is complicated by the fact that clinical practice is as much art as science. *CMAJ*, 1997; **157**: 33–6.

132. Kernick DP. Lies, damned lies, and evidence-based medicine. *Lancet*, 1998; **351**: 1824.

133. Maseri A. Evidence-based medicine: progress but not final solution. *Clin Cardiol*, 1998; **21**: 463–4.

134. Grahame-Smith D. Evidence-based medicine: challenging the orthodoxy. *J Roy Soc Med*, 1998; **91**(Suppl. 35): 7–11.

135. Carr-Hill R. Evidence-based healthcare: flaws in the paradigm? *J Roy Soc Med*, 1998; **91**(Suppl. 35): 12–7.

136. Black D. The limitations of evidence. *J Roy Coll Physicians London*, 1998; **32**: 23–6.

137. Parkin J. Evidence-based practice: the arguments for and against. *Nurs Crit Care*, 1998; **3**: 67–72.

138. Shaugnessy AF, Slawson DC, Becker L. Clinical jazz: harmonizing clinical experience and evidence-based medicine. *J Fam Pract*, 1998; **47**: 425–8.

139. Hampton JR. The limits of evidence-based cardiovascular therapy. *Cardiovasc Drugs Ther*, 1998; **12**: 487–91.

140. Reilly BM, Hart A, Evans AT. Part II. Evidence-based medicine: a passing fancy or the future of primary care? *Dis Mon*,1998; **44**: 370–99.

141. Anderson J. 'Don't confuse me with facts . . .': evidence-based practice confronts reality. *MJA*, 1999; 465–6.

142. Lalwani SI *et al.* Problems with evidence-based medicine. *J Am Assoc Gynecol Laparosc*, 1999; **6**: 237–40.

143. Popay J, Williams G. Qualitative research and evidence-based healthcare. *J Roy Soc Med*, 1998; **91**(Suppl. 35): 32–7.

144. Green J, Britten N. Qualitative research and evidence based medicine. *BMJ*, 1998; **316**: 1230–2.

145. Lecky FE, Driscoll PA. The clinical relevance of observational research. *J Accid Emerg Med*, 1998; **15**: 142–6.

146. Vandenbroucke JP. Observational research and evidence-based medicine: What should we teach young physicians? *J Clin Epidemiol*, 1998; **6**: 467–72.

147. Fowler PB. Evidence-based diagnosis. *J Eval Clin Pract*, 1997; **3**: 153–9.

148. Deeks JJ. Using evaluation of diagnostic tests: understanding their limitations and making the most of available evidence. *Ann Oncol*, 1999; **10**: 761–8.

149. Smeeth L. Time for evidence-based screening? *J Roy Soc Med*, 1998; **91**: 347–8.

150. Steward-Brown SL *et al.* Evidence-based dilemmas in pre-school vision screening. *Arch Dis Child*, 1998; **78**: 406–7.

151. Fletcher SW. Evidence-based screening: what kind of evidence is needed? *ACPJ Club*, 1998; **128**: A12–4.

152. Kerridge I, Lowe M, Henry D. Ethics and evidence-based medicine. *BMJ*, **316**: 1151–3.

153. Pellegrino ED. The ethical use of evidence in biomedicine. *Eval Health Prof*, 1999; **22**: 33–43.

154. Culpeper L, Gilbert TT. Evidence and ethics. *Lancet*, 1999; **356**: 829–31.

155. Bordley DB, Fagan M, Theige D for the APM (Association of Professors of Medicine). Evidence-based medicine: A powerful educational tool for clerkship education. *Am J Med*, 1997, **102**: 427–32.

156. Kenney AF, Hill JE, Mcray CL. Introducing evidence-based medicine into a community family medicine residency. *J Miss State Med Assoc*, 1998; **39**: 441–3.

157. Green ML. Graduate medical education training in clinical epidemiology, critical appraisal, and evidence-based medicine: A critical review of curricula. *Acad Med*, 1999; **74**: 686–94.

158. Haynes B, Haines A. Barriers and bridges to evidence based clinical practice. *BMJ*, 1998; **317**: 273–6.

159. Sackett DL. Evidence-based medicine. *Spine*, 1998; **23**: 1085–6.

160. Kleijnen J, Chalmers I. How to practice and teach evidence-based medicine: role of the Cochrane Collaboration. *Acta Anaesthesiol Scand*, Suppl., 1997; **111**: 231–3.

161. Davidoff F. The future of scientific medicine. *CMAJ*, 1998; **159**: 243–4.

162. Davidoff F. In the teeth of evidence: the curious case of evidence-based medicine. *Mt Sinai J Med*, 1999; **66**: 75–83.

163. Hoey J. The one and only Mrs. Jones. *CMAJ*, 1988; **159**: 241–2.

164. Hurwitz B. Clinical guidelines and the law: advice, guidance or regulation? *J Eval Clin Pract*, 1995; **1**: 49–60.

165. Pelly JE, Newby L, Tito F, Redman S, Adrian AM. Clinical practice guidelines before the law: sword or shield? *Med J Aust*, 1998; **169**: 330–3.

166. Sibbald WJ. Some opinions on the future of evidence-based medicine. *Crit Care Clin*, 1998; **14**: 549–57.

167. Straus SE, McAlister MD. Evidence-based medicine: Past, present, and future. *Annals RCPSC*, 1999; **32**: 260–3.

168. Jenicek M. *Epidemiology, Evidence-Based Medicine, and Evidence-Based Public Health*. Special Lecture at the 2nd Asian-Pacific Congress of Epidemiology and the 8th Scientific Meeting of Japan Epidemiological Association, Tokyo, Japan, January 28–30, 1998.

169. Lohr KN *et al*. Health policy issues and applications for evidence-based medicine and clinical practice guidelines. *Health Policy*, 1998; **46**: 1–19.

170. Feinstein AR. Reflections on reaching a quadricentennial. *J Clin Epidemiol*, 1999; **52**: 1123–9.

171. Hardin WD Jr, Stylianos S, Laly KP. Evidence-based practice in pediatric surgery. *J Pediatr Surg*, 1999; **34**: 908–12; discussion 912–3.

172. Vause S, Macintosh M. Use of prostaglandins to induce labour in women with a cesarean section scar. *BMJ*, 1999; **318**: 1056–8.

173. Browman GP. Essence of evidence-based medicine: A case report. *J Clin Oncol*, 1999; **17**: 1969–73.

174. Vandenbroucke JP. Case reports in an evidence-based world. *J Roy Soc Med*, 1999; **92**: 159–63.

175. Vandenbroucke JP. In defence of case reports and case series. *Ann Int Med*, 2001 (in print).

176. Enkin MW, Jadad AR. Using anecdotal information in evidence-based health care: heresy or necessity? *Ann Oncol*, 1998; **9**: 963–6.

CHAPTER 3

Case studies, casuistics and casuistry in human sciences and medical culture

CHAPTER 3

Case studies, casuistics, and casuistry in human sciences and medical culture

In popular speech and thought, casuistics erroneously means an excessive subtlety and detailing. In contrast, medical casuistics is a process which allows the essential to be extracted from a given patient case or clinical situation

3.1 WHAT IS CASUISTICS?

In medicine, case reporting plays only a limited role in the acquisition of new knowledge. However, its role is very important because it leads to more advanced research. In fact, medical practice often relies on this kind of presentation.

> Today, **casuistics** signifies *'the recording and study of the cases of any disease'*[1]. More precisely, we can define it as an *'observation, analysis and interpretation of clinical cases'*[2]. A **casuist**, then, is a *'practitioner of the study of clinical cases'*[2].

The term 'casuistics' originates from the Latin word *casus* meaning an occurrence, a reality. In lexicography, casuistics refers to the application of general laws or rules to a particular subject or fact. *In general,* casuistics denotes the practice of solving problems by performing certain specific actions based on the general principles and study of similar cases[3]. However, casuistics *as a research method* focuses on the study of special individual cases from which a general rule of action can be derived. Medical casuistics is best defined by the latter explanation.

Several conflicting views of casuistics stem from the field of **casuistry**. In French culture and language, the very same word (*casuistique*) signifies **casuistics, casuistry** and **case studies** (*vide infra*). In English, all these entities are different[4-6].

Over time, casuistry has acquired different meanings in theology, philosophy, economics, administration and business, as well as in popular speech.

3.1.1 Historical comments – casuistry in philosophy, theology and ethics

In opposition to casuistics, **casuistry** is defined as *'a system of rules for distinguishing right from wrong in everyday situations, usually associated with a concept of morality that sees right conduct in terms of obedience to a set of closely defined laws'*. Casuistry was used by the Roman Stoics, Chinese Confucians, Jewish compilers of the Talmud, Muslim commentators of the Qur'an, scholastic philosophers of Medieval Europe and later by Roman Catholic theologians. The fine distinctions employed by some Jesuit casuists compelled their opponents to equate casuistry with specious reasoning[7].

For theologians, casuistry is the part of Christian morality that focuses on states of conscience[8]. A casuist is a theologian who studies morality and offers his or her opinion to help solve cases or states of conscience[9].

Casuistry is also seen as a set of rules that distinguishes right from wrong in daily situations. Such a system is associated with a certain concept of morality that recognizes appropriate behaviour within the context of adherence to a well-defined set of laws. For example, the Talmud in Jewish faith, culture and tradition can be considered an old exercise in casuistry. In contrast, Quebec's Civil Code or similar codes in other parts of the world can be thought of as a modern example in casuistry.

From this historical point of view, health care philosophers or ethicists sometimes identify themselves as *'modern casuists'* [10,11] experienced in the philosophy and theology of morality. This should not be confused with our above-mentioned definition. Health care ethicists assist clinicians in their decisions by applying general arguments of morality to particular individual cases. Should a heart transplant be performed on an elderly patient suffering from another incurable disease? Who should have access to haemodialysis in situations when such access to this technology is limited?

Health care ethicists define casuistry as *'the art of applying abstract principles, paradigms and analogies to particular cases'* [12]. General rules and maxims are not universal and immovable, because they hold true only in relation to the typical situations of the agent and to the circumstances of the action[10].

The direction of inference in medical casuistics is quite different from the direction of inference in theology, philosophy, ethics or business (see Figure 3.1). While the latter apply general concepts to specific cases, medicine, in its will of understanding, starts by studying specific cases and seeks to use them as a basis for general concepts and as the starting point for further research of the problem illustrated by the cases.

A 'case' may be centred not only on an individual patient but also on a particular situation or event. Jonsen and Toulmin[13] describe the controversy surrounding a statement made by Geraldine Ferraro, the first woman to be an American vice-presidential candidate. Although Ms Ferraro was personally opposed to abortion, she declared that the decision to abort should be made by the expectant mother herself. An important discussion

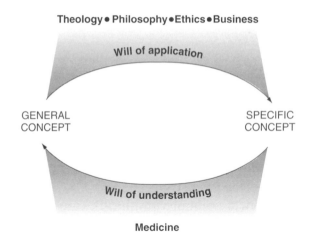

Figure 3.1 – Direction of inference in casuistics

followed on what should prevail: general or universal principles or the particular situation of each and every individual under consideration. It was suggested that an equilibrium between the general and the specific be sought to avoid the challenge of generally accepted values. Because, in this case, the term 'casuistry' could be considered pejorative, its replacement by the French term *'casuistics'* (in French: *'casuistique'*) might be worthy of consideration[13].

Similarly, contemporary medicine relies on the knowledge and mastery of the application of general principles with respect to individuals, communities and specific situations.

Kopelman states, however, and rightly so, that case studies and casuistry do not allow generalizations, and that they risk exposing the casuist researcher to biases favouring a particular individual or situation[14,15].

3.1.2 Casuistics in general understanding and daily life

The excessive detailing of cases, as undertaken by the Jesuits, was not always considered impartial and objective. This led to the image of a casuist as someone who argues a point is too subtle to matter. For many, casuistics or casuistry represented an excessively subtle process of argumentation[8,9].

Clinical casuistics or case reporting is quite a different story, as the rest of this text will illustrate.

CLINICAL CASE REPORTING

3.1.3 General overview of single case concepts and design

Single case studies or single case research designs are often referred to in the general literature as intra-subject-replication designs, n-of-1 research, intensive designs, and so on[16].

This concept stems from a feeling that the advance of science should be based on the integration of what was acquired as information from one individual case (*idiographic approach*) as well as knowledge from a set of cases (*nomothetic approach*)[17].

The more general knowledge is applied to an individual, the more the appropriateness of the qualitative case methods should be considered[17].

A 'case' may be an individual, a given situation, an occurrence or an event in a particular area of daily or professional life. Case studies are carried out in many settings, such as in policy and political science, public administration, community psychology and sociology, organizational and management studies, and city and regional planning[18]. A process, a program, a neighbourhood, an institution or its functioning, or a political, social, cultural or health event can be considered a case in the widest sense of the word. This term's exact meaning is still open to philosophical and conceptual discussion[19].

By stressing these concepts, it should be clear that our clinical case reports are part of a larger philosophical and scientific field than that of medicine and other health sciences.

As for clinical case reporting, the following recurring theme in science fiction movies and literature describes the situation quite well: we are not alone in the universe.

3.1.4 Case studies in administration, management, economics and business

The case method is used to solve a particular case rather than to provide an expanded answer to a more general question. In medicine, we want to work with the data in a patient's chart, to analyse it, and to give direction concerning the best clinical action. In business, the case is a situation to understand and make decisions about to improve a well-defined organization. Typical or extreme cases are analysed in detail as a way to learn how to solve problems[15].

Cases may be *empiric* (stemming from general experience) or *experimental* (the result of a deliberate manipulation).

3.1.5 Case studies in social sciences

Case studies owe their creation not only to medicine, but also to psychology, anthropology and other fields. Social sciences have perhaps made the greatest contributions to the general case study methodology, offering a wide world of learning[19-22] to the public at large.

3.1.5.1 Qualitative research

Contemporary medical research relies heavily on epidemiology and biostatistics. Observations are recorded, summarized, analysed and interpreted with care in order to avoid bias, random errors, or misrepresentation of the events or target groups being studied.

An impressive volume of concepts, methods and thinking has been discussed in the *ad hoc* literature[23-42]. Many experts in the social sciences stress the importance of establishing an equilibrium between what is found in *qualitative research,* i.e. an in-depth study of an individual or situation, and *quantitative research*, which summarizes sets of individual experiences.

Qualitative research was probably best defined by Strauss and Corbin[25] as *'any kind of research that produces findings not arrived at by means of statistical procedures or other means of quantification. It can refer to research about persons' lives, stories, behavior, but also about organizational, functional or social movements, or interactional relationships. Some data may be quantified as with census data but the analysis itself is a qualitative one'.*

In **quantitative research**, series of observations are made, and phenomena are quantified, counted, measured, described, displayed and analysed by statistical methods. Then, the results of these endeavours are applied to the problem as a whole. Biostatistics and epidemiology, which are representative of such undertakings in medicine, have been (and remain) pivotal in decision-oriented medical research. The analysis of disease out-breaks, clinical trials and systematic reviews (meta-analyses) of disease causes or treatment effectiveness are examples of quantita-tive research. In reality, the primary objective of quantitative research is *to provide answers to questions that extend beyond a single observation.*

In **qualitative research**, unique observations are the focus of interest. They are described, studied and analysed in depth. They are not considered as a representative part of a given field before being linked to other observations. The objective of this kind of research is primarily *to understand the case – a single observation itself.*

Research questions can be approached by induction or deduc-tion. **Inductive research** proceeds from observations that serve as a basis for hypotheses and answers. **Deductive research** raises ques-tions first, then gathers observations relevant to the problem, and confirms or rejects hypotheses 'free from or independent of the material under study'.

Quantitative research is both inductive and deductive. Epi-demiologists, for obvious reasons, prefer the deductive compo-nent. Qualitative research is mostly inductive by definition. It is driven not by hypotheses, but by questions, issues and a search for patterns[43]. Classification is therefore its purpose.

We agree with Pope and Mays[44] that the focus of qualitative research is *'what is a given observation (X, case)?'* Quantitative research, however, counts *'how many Xs?'*

Let us remember that qualitative research principles are not foreign to medicine. Medical histories, psychiatric interviews and the study of index cases (i.e. those that lead to quantitative research) of disease outbreaks or of new phenomena (poisoning, infection etc.) possess characteristics of qualitative research.

Obviously, equilibrium between quantitative and qualitative research is both necessary and beneficial[25,45–48], not only in social sci-ences but in health sciences as well.

3.1.5.2 Concept of a 'case'

The definition of the term 'case', which some[45] also refer to as 'site', remains slightly unclear[49]. It may[23,50] include the following (with examples given in parentheses):

- a person (in medicine and nursing);
- an event or situation (marital discord, strike);
- an action (spousal abuse) – and
- its remedy (consulting and its result);
- a programme (home care for chronic patients);
- a time period (baby boomers era);
- a critical incident (hostage taking);
- a small group (homeless people);
- a department (within an organization);
- an organization itself (company, political party);
- a community (people living on welfare, suburbanites etc.).

One 'case' may be studied and presented in different ways. For example, we can examine the Watergate case by focusing on the men behind the case, the event itself (a break-in at the office of a political party), or the attempts made to cover it up[18].

3.1.5.3 Case studies

> For Rothe[50] *'The term "case study" comes from the tradition of legal, medical and psychological research, where it refers to a detailed analysis of an individual case, and explains the dynamics and pathology of a given disease, crime or disorder. The assumption underlying case studies is that we can properly acquire knowledge of a phenomenon from intense exploration of a single example'.*

Case studies can be qualitative (based on a search for a meaning) or quantitative (based on some kind of measurement).

A clinical examination is both qualitative (history taking, psychiatric evaluation) and quantitative (anthropometry, examination of vital functions etc.).

In contrast, a social worker focuses more on qualitative information through three types of case studies[51]:

1. In an *intrinsic case study*, a better understanding of a case is sought (e.g. why did parents abandon their child?).

2. In an *instrumental case study*, a better understanding of the problem represented by the case or the refinement of an underlying theory of the problem is sought (e.g. parental child neglect).

3. A *collective case study* is not an epidemiological exploration (no target groups, no denominators etc.), but rather an extension of an instrumental case study of several cases. Its concept resembles that of case series reports, as we will see in Chapter 5.

Some researchers may study only selected phenomena that illustrate the case[52] adequately. Others may choose a *monographic study* that is as detailed and complete as possible. The nature of this kind of research is inductive[54].

> Casuistics in medicine and social sciences both agree that case studies do not permit generalizations. However, if a case study brings results contrary to previous experience, generalizations from previous experiences should be reviewed.

3.1.6 Other uses of single cases in biology and human sciences

In experimental psychology and physiology, studies of individual cases and sets of cases are undertaken to acquire new knowledge. In a quantitative study of multiple cases, the results obtained apply to groups or communities that are represented by the subjects being studied. They do not necessarily apply to each and every particular case (individual) under study.

To better understand what happens in a particular case, a *single case experimental design* is used[18,50,55,56]. This type of study should lead to improved decisions related to a particular individual or experimental subject studied. The *n*-of-1 studies in medicine (see Section 3.1.7) have a similar conceptual basis.

3.1.7 Return of qualitative research to medicine, nursing and public health

Qualitative research, like any other scientific concept, technique or method, isn't immune to the ebb and flow of information from one field to another.

In the past, experience gathered from the study of single individuals in medicine, psychology or nursing was used, modified and expanded in social sciences, business, finance, administration, law and the military. In these other areas, the 'case' concept extended beyond an individual to encompass situations, states or events. The resulting enriched methodology has now returned to the health sciences.

3.1.7.1 Qualitative approach in case research

Recently, the *BMJ* introduced its readers to qualitative research in health sciences, and in medicine in particular, by means of an excellent reader-friendly group of articles[44,57-63] that have appeared subsequently in book form[64].

As a result of impressive papers based on qualitative research, medical authors and readers now face increasing pressure with regards to the content and form of their written work. Greenhalgh[65] has suggested ways to read and understand *'papers that go beyond numbers'*. Hence, qualitative research has slowly joined the mainstream of findings in health sciences.

Family medicine calls for qualitative research[66]. Nursing[48,67-70], as a health profession and field of health research, has a longer history of qualitative research, for which it traditionally reserved a place of significant importance.

In health administration, medical care organization and health services research, case studies are used in their expanded sense[63]. Incentives arising from the removal from insurance of *in vitro* fertilization[71], the consequences of the introduction of public funding for midwifery[72], or patients' unmet expectations of care[73,74] can all be cited as examples.

3.1.7.2 Quantitative approach in case research

Patients as 'cases'

In the same spirit that encouraged experimental research in psychology, experimental research and clinical trials involving a single individual (**n-of-1 study, single case study**)[75-80] have been presented to physicians as a means of selecting the most appropriate treatment for a particular patient.

In this type of case research, instead of randomizing patients (there is only one anyway), treatment modalities are randomized. Multiple spells of disease of short duration with short remissions between them are particularly suitable for such an evaluation (angina, tension headache, migraine etc.). This approach can help physicians make decisions in individual cases. It can also be considered in cases where other types of clinical trials are impossible, for whatever reason, or in cases where the results of classical trials do not apply to the patient in question[75].

Situations as 'cases'

A 'case' may be a question to answer or, most commonly, a controversial[80] problem to clarify. For example, it might be of interest to better understand the effects of dietary intake or drug control on blood cholesterol levels. *Meta-analysis* as a kind of systematic review of evidence relating to the 'case' is generally very helpful in assessing these situations. In a wide sense, meta-analysis is a 'case study'.

In reality, the study of a clinical case (patient) should lead to the re-evaluation of acquired knowledge. It should offer something new, particularly in cases where other approaches cannot be used in an unbiased way and without a preconceived idea of the problem. The study of a clinical case must therefore be a 'systematic review' of evidence, even if the evidence is relatively weak at this level.

In the narrower area of an *'acquaintance with particulars'*[81], the study and reporting of clinical cases as medical casuistics remain the core practice of repeated daily use, and the most frequent method of qualitative research. The rest of this book is devoted to this subject.

3.2 MEDICAL CASUISTICS AS AN ENTRY LINK IN THE CHAIN OF EVIDENCE

Recent impressive developments in medical research based on increasingly large samples of individuals have made the study of single clinical cases a kind of neglected orphan of medical research rather than a necessity of daily clinical routine. Perhaps the opposite should occur.

Improved selection, observation, analysis, interpretation and reporting of a clinical case is a 'missing link' in the acquisition of medical knowledge.

Any advanced research should and often does begin with the study of one of several index cases. Figure 3.2 illustrates the situation.

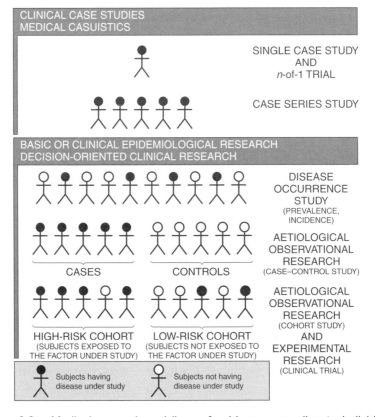

Figure 3.2 – Medical research and lines of evidence according to individuals involved

Most often, we record the first case(s), i.e. the index case(s), of an interesting and important phenomenon. An **index case** is defined in medical genetics as an *'original patient (propositus or proband) which provides the stimulus for study of other members of the family, to ascertain a possible genetic factor in causation of the presenting condition'* [4]. By extension, any first case that triggers a more advanced investigation is an index case.

First cases of vomiting and diarrhoea might be index cases of a food poisoning outbreak, leading to the investigation of an epidemic. In toxicology and environmental medicine, the first occurrences of respiratory problems led to an elucidation of the role of toxic fumes in silo filler's disease. In the area of new medical technology, the first unexpected deaths of some users of an insulin pump were index cases leading to the surveillance of the problem, the evaluation of the risk factors, and ultimately to the modification of the criteria for initiating pump use[82]. Any unexpected beneficial effect of a drug in situations other than those for which it was primarily intended forms an index case for an *ad hoc* clinical trial. As two examples, Minoxidil® was found to be a hair growth stimulant and the intended use of Viagra® changed from the treatment of hypertension.

Figure 3.2 outlines the cascading steps of a medical investigation:

Step 1. Case studies are the starting point in the development of a portrait of disease occurrence, its treatment or outcomes, based on epidemiological surveillance and other means.

Step 2. Linking cases to one or more control groups (unaffected individuals) means that a case–control search for causes will be performed. A group of unaffected individuals is added to a set of cases.

Step 3. Comparing exposed and unexposed individuals produces a cohort study, be it observational or experimental (clinical trial). Cases will develop or improve depending on exposure (drug, poison etc.).

If a case study means 'noticing the problem', such noticing must take place at other steps of the cascade as well. Today, the methodology of case studies and reports must be as refined and sophisticated as that of case–control studies or clinical trials.

In addition, because a case study is a first link in the chain of evidence, other steps do not necessarily have to follow for some time. A single case or case series (with all their inherent limitations) may long remain the only evidence available. If that happens, single cases or case series must provide the best evidence in their contexts. Long ago, generations of faithful were naturally curious about the Old and New Testament's 'case reports' of various miracles and heavenly events. To this day, like the Immaculate Conception and Ezekiel's bones, they remain the only cases universally known.

If we are reasonably well trained and experienced in aetiological observational research and clinical trials, should we not master equally well the methodology of clinical case study and reporting?

3.3 IS THERE A NEED FOR BETTER TRAINING IN CLINICAL CASE STUDIES – AND HOW IMPORTANT ARE CLINICAL CASE REPORTS TODAY?

3.3.1 Medical casuistics

Case studies and qualitative research share many characteristics. As soon as a patient enters a medical office or hospital, the attending physician, often without knowing it, uses one or several components of qualitative research. Clinimetrics are a quantitative counterpart in the study and assessment of clinical cases.

Moreover, qualitative aspects of care and research differentiate such disciplines as family medicine or psychiatry. Psychoanalysis *per se* has been a kind of qualitative research since Josef Breuer and Sigmund Freud's 'Case of Anna O (Bertha Pappenheim)'.

We are all aware that a better understanding of many previously poorly known phenomena was made possible by the relevant observation and reporting of index cases. Examples are the case of maple syrup disease, isoimmunization in pregnancy, acquired immunodeficiency syndrome and multiple personality disorder, to name just a few. Some clinical case reports pertaining to these illnesses have become landmark articles in medicine.

William Osler knew that the best training in medicine, as a whole, is that which focuses on individual cases and bedside care[83]: *'The amphitheatre clinic, the ward and dispensary classes are but bastard substitutes for a system which makes the medical student himself help in the work . . . put him (i.e. the student) behind a case. Ask any physician of twenty years' standing how he has become proficient in his art, and he will reply that (what) he learned in the schools was totally different from the medicine he learned at the bedside. Medicine is learned by the bedside and not in the classroom'.* If such experiences are not properly recorded and shared through a clinical case report, for instance, the most valuable part of clinical wisdom will be lost.

As Kathryn Montgomery Hunter stated[21]: *'Despite the refinements of clinical epidemiology and the study of decision making, the careful construction and interpretation of the individual case remains essential to learning and remembering in clinical medicine. Medical education cultivates and clinical practice refines clinical judgement. Medicine, then, is practised casuistically somewhere between the forest of textbooks and a thicket of (algorithm) trees. Narrative is the ultimate device of casuistry in medicine (as in theology and law), which enables practitioners who share its diagnostic and therapeutic world view to fit general principles to the single case and to achieve a degree of generalization that is both practicable and open to change'.*

> If clinical case study and reporting regroups the qualitative finesse of observation, the rigor of measurement and classification of clinimetrics, and the pragmatic need for ensuing medical decisions, then medical casuistics is not only *'the recording and study of cases of any disease'* [1], but also **the art of choosing, gathering, structuring and conveying pragmatic information about relevant clinical cases. It must lead to a better understanding of a given health problem and improved clinical decisions. It should focus on the reduction of information to be gathered, rather than on the accumulation and detailing of a given volume of data.**
>
> Clinical medicine needs direction with regards to what to do with particular patients or groups of

patients. Hence, *'The more a programme aims at individual outcomes, the greater the appropriateness of qualitative case methods. The more a programme emphasizes common outcomes for all participants, the greater may be the appropriateness of standardized quantitative measures of performance and change'* [17].

3.3.2 Specific situations and questions as cases

For some, a case study should evaluate only controversial situations. A 'case' then becomes a problem to be solved. As an example, the role of dietary intake or drugs on blood cholesterol levels can be studied. Meta-analysis can be used to clarify the problem.

In the same spirit, a unique case study should incite the revision of acquired knowledge. It should offer something new, for example an answer to a question that cannot be obtained by other types of studies or means. **Therefore, shouldn't a systematic review of literature or a meta-analysis be seen as a kind of 'case study'?**

Such a widened concept of medical casuistics is based on new paradigms and on the revision of old ones that focused on one particular case or on several cases taken from hospital or community settings.

3.4 CONCLUSIONS

Multiple cases call for a balance between qualitative and quantitative research in medicine and other health sciences.

A 'case' may be an individual patient, for example, whose unexpectedly localized aneurysm rupture is associated with some unexpected clinical manifestations possibly requiring some special emergency and surgical care.

A situation may be a 'case'. Recently, an in-flight emergency was reported[84,85]. A passenger developed a tension pneumothorax requiring an improvised chest drain on board an aircraft. The problem was solved by using improvised material including a modified coat hanger as a trocar, a bottle of mineral water with two holes created in its cap as an underwater seal drain, and five star brandy as a disinfectant for the introducer. The treatment was successful and a proposal for dealing with future similar air transportation emergencies was published in the medical press.

Case reports should not simply be centred on presenting unusual cases. They should lead to the surveillance of rare cases, to the explanation of the underlying mechanisms and treatment of cases, and to the direction required for future research[86]. They should also generate new hypotheses although these hypotheses cannot be confirmed by single cases.

A specific methodology must be taught and put into practice as outlined in the next chapter.

Is this really necessary? Absolutely!

Calls for qualitative research abound in various specialties[81,87–90], as do calls for better clinical case presentations[91–94] because they play an ever-increasing role in various clinical training programs and are subject to evaluation[95–102]. Moreover, editors of medical journals now provide more detailed indications of their expectations with regards to clinical case reporters[103,104] and their reports.

REFERENCES

1. *Mosby's Medical Dictionary*, 5th Edition. St Louis: Mosby, 1998.
2. Jenicek M. *Casuistique Médicale. Bien Présenter un Cas Clinique.* (Medical Casuistics. Good Clinical Case Reporting.) St Hyacinthe and Paris: Edisem and Maloine, 1997.
3. Vereecke L-G. Casuistique. pp. 61–62 in: *Encyclopaedia Universalis*, Corpus 5. Paris: Encyclopaedia Universalis, Éditeur à Paris, 1989.
4. Dorland WAN. *Dorland's Illustrated Medical Dictionary*, 27th Edition. Edited by EJ Taylor. Philadelphia: WB Saunders, 1988.
5. *Collins Robert French/English English/French Dictionary (Unabridged)*, 3rd Edition. Glasgow: Harper Collins, 1993.
6. *Dictionnaire de Médecine Flammarion*, 4th Edition. Paris: Flammarion, 1991.
7. *Encyclopedia Britannica*, 15th Edition. Chicago: Encyclopedia Britannica, 1992.
8. *Dictionnaire de Français 'Plus' à l'Usage des Francophones d'Amérique*. Montreal: CEC (Centre Educatif et Culturel Inc.), 1988.
9. *Dictionnaire Encyclopédique Larousse*. Paris: Librairie Larousse, 1979.
10. Jonsen AR. Casuistry and clinical ethics. *Theor Med*, 1986; **7**: 65–74.
11. Jonsen AR. Casuistry as methodology in clinical ethics. *Theor Med*, 1991; **12**: 295–307.

12. Arras JD. Getting down to cases: the revival of casuistry in bioethics. *J Med Phil*, 1991; **16**: 29–51.

13. Jonsen AR, Toulmin S. *The Abuse of Casuistry. A History of Moral Reasoning.* Berkeley: University of California Press, 1988.

14. Kopelman LM. Case method and casuistry: The problem of bias. *Theor Med*, 1994; **15**: 21–37.

15. Pagès R. Cas (méthode des), pp. 34–37 in *Encyclopaedia Universalis*, Corpus 5. Paris, Encyclopaedia Universalis, Éditeur à Paris, 1989.

16. Kazdin AE. *Single-Case Research Designs. Methods for Clinical and Applied Settings.* New York: Oxford University Press, 1980.

17. Patton MQ. *Qualitative Evaluation Methods.* Beverly Hills: Sage Publications, 1980.

18. Yin RK. *Case Study Research. Design and Methods.* Newbury Park: Sage Publications, 1988.

19. *What Is a Case? Exploring the Foundations of Social Inquiry.* Edited by CC Ragin and HS Becker. Cambridge: Cambridge University Press, 1992.

20. Barlow DH, Hersen M. *Single Case Experimental Designs. Strategies for Studying Behavior Change.* New York: Pergamon Press, 1984.

21. Hunter Montgomery K. A science of individuals: medicine and casuistry. *J Med Phil*, 1989; **14**: 193–212.

22. Stake R. *The Art of Case Study Research.* Thousand Oaks: Sage, 1995.

23. Miles M, Huberman AM. *Qualitative Data Analysis: A Sourcebook of New Methods.* Newbury Park: Sage, 1989.

24. Guba EG, Lincoln YS. *Fourth Generation Evaluation.* Newbury Park: Sage, 1989.

25. Strauss A, Corbin J. *Basics of Qualitative Research. Grounded Theory Procedures and Techniques.* Newbury Park: Sage Publications, 1990.

26. Tesch R. *Qualitative Research: Analysis Types and Software Tools.* New York: The Falmer Press, 1990.

27. Patton MQ. *Qualitative Evaluation and Research Methods.* Newbury Park: Sage, 1990.

28. Crabtree BF, Miller WL. *Doing Qualitative Research.* Newbury Park: Sage, 1992.

29. Wolcott HF. *Transforming Qualitative Data.* Thousand Oaks: Sage, 1994.

30. Guba EG, Lincoln YS. Competing paradigms in qualitative research, pp. 105–119 in: *Handbook of Qualitative Research.* Edited by NK Denzin and YS Lincoln. Thousand Oaks: Sage, 1994.

31. Creswell JW. *Research Design. Qualitative & Quantitative Approaches.* Thousand Oaks: Sage, 1994.

32. Miller WL, Crabtree BF. Clinical research, pp. 340–352 in: *Handbook of Qualitative Research.* Edited by NK Denzin and YS Lincoln. Thousand Oaks: Sage, 1994.

33. Adler PA, Adler P. Observational techniques, pp. 377–392 in: *Handbook of Qualitative Research.* Edited by NK Denzin and YS Lincoln. Thousand Oaks: Sage, 1994.

34. Fontana A, Frey JH. Interviewing. The art of science, pp. 361–376 in: *Handbook of Qualitative Research.* Edited by NK Denzin and YS Lincoln. Thousand Oaks: Sage, 1994.

35. Marshall C, Rossman CB. *Designing Qualitative Research*, 2nd Edition. Newbury Park: Sage, 1994.

36. Rubin HJ, Rubin IS. *Qualitative Interviewing. The Art of Hearing Data*. Thousand Oaks: Sage, 1995.

37. Weitzman EA, Miles MB. *A Software Sourcebook: Computer Programs for Qualitative Data Analysis*. Thousand Oaks: Sage, 1995.

38. Mason J. *Qualitative Researching*. London: Sage, 1996.

39. Kvale S. *Interviews: An Introduction to Qualitative Research Interviewing*. Thousand Oaks: Sage, 1996.

40. Coffey A, Atkinson P. *Making Sense of Qualitative Data*. Thousand Oaks: Sage, 1997.

41. Schwandt TS. *Qualitative Inquiry: A Dictionary of Terms*. Thousand Oaks: Sage, 1997.

42. Creswell JW. *Qualitative Inquiry and Research Design. Choosing Among Five Traditions*. Thousand Oaks: Sage, 1998.

43. Patton MQ. *How to Use Qualitative Methods in Evaluation*. Newbury Park: Sage Publications, 1987.

44. Pope C, Mays N. Reaching the parts others cannot reach: an introduction to qualitative methods in health and health services research. *BMJ*, 1995; **311**: 42–5.

45. Denzin NK, Lincoln YS. Introduction. Entering the field of qualitative research (Chapter 1), pp. 1–17 in: *Handbook of Qualitative Research*. Edited by NK Denzin and YS Lincoln. Thousand Oaks: Sage, 1994.

46. Miles MB, Huberman AM. *Qualitative Data Analysis: A Sourcebook of New Methods*. Beverly Hills: Sage Publications, 1984.

47. Verhoef MJ, Casebeer AL. Broadening horizons: Integrating quantitative and qualitative research. *Can J Infect Dis*, 1997; **8**: 65–6.

48. Dzurec LC, Abraham IL. The nature of inquiry: Linking quantitative and qualitative research. *Adv Nurs Sci*, 1993; **16**: 73–9.

49. Ragin CC. Introduction: Cases of 'What is a case?', pp. 1–17 in: *What is a Case? Exploring the Foundation of Social Inquiry*. Edited by CC Ragin and HS Becker. Cambridge: Cambridge University Press, 1992.

50. Rothe JP. *Qualitative Research. A Practical Guide*. Heidelberg and Toronto: RCI/PDE Publications, 1993.

51. Stake RE. Case studies (Chapter 14), pp. 236–247 in: *Handbook of Qualitative Research*. Edited by NK Denzin and YS Lincoln. Thousand Oaks: Sage Publications, 1994.

52. Aday LA. *Designing and Conducting Health Surveys. A Comprehensive Guide*. San Francisco and London: Jossey-Bass Publishers, 1989.

53. Patton MQ. *How to Use Qualitative Methods in Evaluation*. Newbury Park: Sage Publications, 1987.

54. Yin RK. *Applications of Case Studies Research*. Thousand Oaks: Sage Publications, 1993.

55. Kazdin AE. *Single-Case Research Designs. Methods for Clinical and Applied Settings*. New York: Oxford University Press, 1982.

56. Barlow DH, Hersen M. *Single Case Experimental Designs. Strategies for Studying Behavior Change*. New York: Pergamon Press, 1984.
57. Jones R. Why do qualitative research? It should begin to close the gap between the sciences of discovery and implementation. *BMJ*, 1995; **311**: 2.
58. Mays N, Pope C. Rigour and qualitative research. *BMJ*, 1995; **311**: 109–12.
59. Mays N, Pope C. Observational methods in health care settings. *BMJ*, 1995; **311**: 182–4.
60. Britten N. Qualitative interview in medical research. *BMJ*, 1995; **311**: 251–3.
61. Kitzinger J. Introducing focus groups. *BMJ*, 1995; **311**:299–302.
62. Jones J, Hunter D. Consensus methods for medical and health services research. *BMJ*, 1995; **311**: 376–80.
63. Keen J, Packwood T. Case study evaluation. *BMJ*, 1995; **311**: 444–6.
64. *Qualitative Research in Health Care*. Edited by N Mays and C Pope. London: BMJ Publishing Group, 1996.
65. Greenhalgh T. Papers that go beyond numbers (qualitative research) (Chapter 11), pp. 151–162 in: *How to Read a Paper. The Basics of Evidence Based Medicine*. London: BMJ Publishing Group, 1997.
66. Burkett GL, Godkin MA. Qualitative research in family medicine. *J Family Practice*, 1983; **16**:625–6.
67. Goodwin LD, Goodwin WL. Qualitative *vs.* quantitative research or qualitative *and* quantitative research? *Nurs Res*, 1984; **33**: 378–80.
68. Skodol Wilson H. Qualitative studies: from observations to explanations. *J Nurs Admin*, 1985; **15**: 8–10 (May).
69. Meier P, Pugh EJ. The case study: A viable approach to clinical research. *Res Nurs Health*, 1986; **9**: 195–202.
70. Sandelowski M. One of the liveliest number: The case orientation of qualitative research. *Res Nurs Health*, 1996; **19**: 525–9.
71. Giacomini M, Hurley J, Stoddart G, Schneider D, West S. When tinkering is too much. A case study of incentives arising from Ontario's deinsurance of *in vitro* fertilization. Paper 96-10. Hamilton: McMaster University Centre for Health Economics and Policy Analysis, Working Paper Series, August 1996.
72. Giacomini M, Peters M. The introduction of public funding for midwifery in Ontario: Interpreting the meaning of the financial incentives. Paper 96-9. Hamilton: McMaster University Centre for Health Economics and Policy Analysis, Working Paper Series, August 1996.
73. Kravitz RL, Callahan EJ, Paterniti D, Antonius D, Dunham M, Lewis CE, Prevalence and sources of patients' unmet expectations for care. *Ann Intern Med*, 1996; **125**: 730–7.
74. Inui TS. The virtue of qualitative *and* quantitative research. *Ann Intern Med*, 1996; **125:** 770–1.
75. Gyuatt G, Sackett D, Taylor DW, Chong J, Roberts R, Pugsley S. Determining optimal therapy – randomized trials in individual patients. *N Engl J Med*, 1986; **314**: 889–92.
76. Guyatt G, Sackett D, Adachi J, Roberts R, Chong J, Rosenbloom D, Keller J. A

clinician's guide for conducting randomized trials in individual patients. *CMAJ*, 1988; **139**: 497–503.

77. Single Case Studies. Proceedings from a symposium in Oslo, 14–15 March 1987. Edited by H Petersen. *Scand J Gastroenterol*, 1988; **23**: Suppl 147, 1–48.

78. Guyatt GH, Keller JL, Jaeschke R, Rosenblooom D, Adachi JD, Newhouse MT. The *n*-of-1 randomized controlled clinical trial: Clinical usefulness. Our three year experience. *Ann Intern Med*, 1990; **112**: 293–9.

79. Hodgson M. *N*-of-one clinical trials. The practice of environmental and occupational medicine. *J Occup Environ Med*, 1993; **35**: 375–80.

80. West R. Assessment of evidence versus consensus or prejudice. *J Epidemiol Comm Med*, 1992; **46**: 321–2.

81. McWhinney IR. 'An acquaintance with particulars'. *Fam Med*, 1989; **21**: 296–8.

82. Thacker SB, Berkelman RL. Surveillance of medical technologies. *J Public Health Policy*, 1986; **7**: 363–77.

83. *Counsels and Ideals from the Writings of William Osler & Selected Aphorisms*. Compiled and edited by CNB Camac (Counsels and Ideals) and LJ Beam (Selected Aphorisms). Birmingham: The Classics of Medicine Library, 1985.

84. Wallace WA. Managing in flight emergencies. A personal account. *BMJ*, 1995; **311**: 374–6.

85. Wallace WA, Wong T, O'Bichere A, Ellis BW. Discussion, *BMJ*, 1995; **311**: 375–6.

86. Fletcher RH, Fletcher SW, Wagner EH. Studying cases (Chapter 10), pp. 208–212 in: *Clinical Epidemiology. The Essentials*. Baltimore: Williams & Wilkins, 1996.

87. McWhinney IR. Changing models: The impact of Kuhn's theory on medicine. *Family Practice*, 1983; **1**: 3–8.

88. Rainsberry RPN. Values, paradigms and research in family medicine. *Family Practice*, 1986; **3**: 209–15.

89. Naess MH, Malterud K. Patients' stories: science, clinical facts or fairy tales? *Scand J Prim Health Care*, 1994; **12**: 59–64.

90. Shafer A, Fish MP. A call for narrative: The patient's story and anesthesia training. *Literature and Medicine*, 1994 (Spring); **13**: 124–42.

91. Engel GL. The deficiencies of the case presentation as a method of clinical teaching. *N Engl J Med*, 1971; **284**: 20–4.

92. Allen LC, Bunting PS. Postdoctoral training in clinical chemistry: Laboratory training aspects. *Clin Biochem*, 1995; **28**: 481–97.

93. Hormbrey P, Todd BS, Mansfield CD, Skinner DV. A survey of teaching and the use of clinical guidelines in accident and emergency departments. *J Accid Emerg Med*, 1996; **13**: 129–33.

94. Haddad D, Robertson KJ, Cockburn F, Helms P, McIntosh N, Olver RE. What is core? Guidelines for the core curriculum in paediatrics. *Med Educ*, 1997; **31**: 354–8.

95. Klos M, Reuler JB, Nardone DA, Girard DE. An evaluation of trainee performance in the case presentation. *J Med Educ*, 1983; **58**: 432–4.

96. Kihm JT, Brown JT, Divine GW, Linzer M. Quantitative analysis of the outpatient oral case presentation: Piloting a method. *J Gen Intern Med*, 1991; **6**: 233–6.

97. Gennis VM, Gennis MA. Supervision in the outpatient clinic: Effects on teaching and patient care. *J Gen Intern Med*, 1993; **8**: 378–80.

98. Templeton B, Selarnick HS. Evaluating consultation psychiatry residents. *Gen Hosp Psychiatry*, 1994; **16**: 326–34.

99. Raik B, Fein O, Wachspress S. Measuring the use of the population perspective on internal medicine attending rounds. *Acad Med*, 1995; **70**: 1047–9.

100. Greenberg LW, Getson PR. Assessing student performance on a pediatric clerkship. *Arch Pediatr Adolesc Med*, 1996; **150**: 1209–12.

101. Elliot DL, Hickam DH. How do faculty evaluate student's case presentations? *Teach Learn Med*, 1997; **9**: 261–3.

102. Bass EB, Fortin AH, Morrison G, Wills S, Mumford LM, Goroll AH. National survey of clerkship directors in internal medicine on the competencies that should be addressed in the medicine core clerkship. *Am J Med*, 1997; **102**: 564–71.

103. Squires BP. Case reports: What editors want from authors and peer reviewers. *CMAJ*, 1989; **141**: 379–80.

104. Squires BP, Elmslie TJ. Reports of case series: What editors expect from authors and peer reviewers. *CMAJ*, 1990; **142**: 1205–6.

CHAPTER 4

Reporting routine clinical cases lacking in 'scientific value'

CHAPTER 4

Reporting routine clinical cases lacking in 'scientific value'

4.1 REPORTING ROUTINE CLINICAL CASES LACKING IN SCIENTIFIC VALUE IN A MEDICAL SETTING

Routine clinical case reports are divided into three categories:

- Case studies with follow-up in progress. A case report is a **progress report** prepared for others, usually in a ward setting. **Morning reports** or **admission reports** are usually included within this category.

- Closed cases where the course, management, outcomes, and future plans are outlined. **Discharge summaries** are a good example of this type of report.
- Case **reports** used outside the hospital **for non-medical purposes**. These include compensation claims in occupational medicine and tort litigations.

In all these situations, evidence is weighed throughout the case reporting process.

4.1.1 Routine reporting of a clinical case in wards: morning and admission reports in medicine, surgery and psychiatry

Even the most routine, 'uninteresting' (boring for some) case report should be presented as a meaningful, organized, **critically assessed topic**[1] for EBM protagonists[1] and its practitioners also.

Let us take a clinical example: a man brings his 35-year-old single nulliparous female companion to the hospital emergency department because she is suffering from abdominal pain. She is agitated, crying and not very communicative. At this point, no evaluation has yet taken place.

Based on intuition, previous experience and learned knowledge, the attending emergency care specialist might consider, even before examining the patient, that the abdominal pain she is suffering from is caused by one of the following: appendicitis, extra uterine pregnancy, incipient spontaneous abortion, endometriosis, pelvic inflammatory disease, mesenteric lymphadenitis or infarction, food poisoning, another infection (parasitic, etc.) or intoxication. The emergency care specialist might also consider whether the patient is having a hysterical reaction to a recent couple dispute or feeling the effects of depression, an acute reaction to drug abuse, or injury by accident or by spousal abuse.

Once this patient is examined and evaluated, how should her case be reported?

The sequence of information sought and given in a standard admission or progress clinical report is certainly familiar to most readers, although it may vary from one clinical environment and culture to another.

A **routine clinical case report in medicine or surgery** should have the following components:

- **Patient identification and demographic characteristics** (age, sex, occupation, etc.).
- **Chief complaint** and **reason for admission**.
- **Complaint history** and the history of possibly related present and past health problems. Such a history is based on deductive reasoning about patient problem causes.
- **Patient history** (medical, surgical, personal health, family, social, occupational, alternative medicine exposure, lay care, risk exposure from all relevant sources, health maintenance).
- **Patient views**[1], such as their ideas about the nature of their problem, **concerns, expectations**, and **values** given to their state, its management and future. N.B. An important addition emphasized by the 'human face' of EBM.
- **Physical examination**, i.e. relevant findings.
- **Paraclinical evaluation** (laboratory, imaging, and other technology dependent results).
- **Psychiatric assessment** if relevant and necessary for a joint medical, surgical, and psychiatric evaluation and management of the patient (see below).
- **'Impression'**, i.e. a working (provisional) diagnosis.
- **Immediate treatment and care plan** and **orders** including alternative strategies if the preferred option will not work, whatever the reason might be.
- **Differential diagnostic work-up plan**.
- **Prognosis and priority classification** for immediate and future clinical management.

As we can see, a 'modern' case report includes three additional main elements:

- Exposure to **non-traditional treatments**, such as herbal medicines, that often have their own therapeutic and adverse effects. Also, for the same reason, **other diagnostic and therapeutic methods** of treatment like chiropractic and acupuncture must be taken into account.
- **Patient preferences** should be considered and become part of clinical decision making and case management.
- Review of **alternative case management strategies**, no matter what their underlying cause.

The objective of such a morning (admission) report is to give essential information about the case, to reproduce the clinical work-up and step by step reasoning of the attending physician, and to give clues for future clinical and paraclinical management of this case as well as related administrative requirements: admission, social service evaluation, etc. Anyone who takes over the subsequent care of the patient should be able to continue without having to start again from scratch.

In a 'modern' clinical case report, the emphasis must be placed on alternative strategies for the patient management plan as well as on the justification for these strategies. All health professionals should be interested in alternative strategies in situations of:

- Diagnostic error and its consequences.
- No effect of treatment.
- Unexpected and adverse reactions to treatment.
- Choice of other patient management options in situations well-suited to decision analysis.
- Patient migration from one service or care site to another.

A **routine case report in psychiatry** covers several additional topics of particular relevance to the specialty. The following set of components is based on Boston (see Carlat[2]) and Montreal (Prelevic – personal communication, author) experience and current practice of writing up the results of the interview:

CLINICAL CASE REPORTING

- **Identifying data**   Patient characteristics and location within the context of social and cultural norms.
- **Referring party**   Is the patient seeking help actively or involuntarily (sent by a third party (judge, police, family)? In involuntary patients specify the reason for assessment: chief complaint or other?
- **Chief complaint**   Patient's verbatim statement.
- **Source of information**   Patient, company or relatives, interview with patient, review of patients charts (local and including those from other places if necessary), case discussion with medical, surgical, and/or psychiatric staff, other.
- **History of present illness**   History of existing psychiatric disorder and history of present crisis (including the premorbid level of functioning).
- **Past and present psychiatric and developmental history**   Including substance use and abuse, hospitalizations, care, medications, electroconvulsive therapy, psychotherapy, family, education, work, intimate relationships, present activities and interactions.
- **General medical history**   As in a general medical and surgical report but focused on elements relevant for the psychiatric problem under study and care, i.e. for psychiatric diagnosis and treatment.
- **Family, social, and medical history**   Relevant for psychotherapy considerations (social and psy-psychiatric history), mental

	disorder aetiology, links to organic disorders, and foreseeable pharmacological treatment following the incoming diagnosis (medical history); genogram.
• **Mental status examination**	Distinct coverage of appearance and behaviour; state of consciousness; orientation; mood and affect; psychomotor activity; speech; memory; perception, thought content and process; cognitive functions; intelligence; judgement; insight; suicidal and homicidal ideation, death wishes (risk assessment); fears, preoccupations and concerns.
• **Assessment**	Summary recapitulation of the overall clinical picture (including dynamics of illness, course) and discussion of differential diagnosis. Is the diagnosis built on patient's subjective elements, on physician's interpretation or both? Does the diagnosis mean good or bad prognosis?
• **DSM* IV diagnosis**	Particularly important for any litigation (insurance or other): Main psychiatric diagnosis (**Axis I**), personality disorders and mental retardation (**Axis II**), relevant medical conditions related to psychiatric diagnosis and those affecting patient's current functioning (**Axis III**), psychosocial problems poten-

tially aggravating patient's mental disorder(s) (**Axis IV**), and degree of impairment of patient's psychological, social and occupational functioning by the problem under this evaluation and clinical management by the GAF** numeric scale (**Axis V**).

- **Treatment plan ('orders')** — Including planned diagnostic work-up (testing), medication, other therapy, security measures for both the patient and his/her surroundings, referrals to other specialties' evaluation and plans, social evaluation, management, and care of the patient and his or her extramural environment; alternative plans.

---

* Diagnostic and Statistical Manual of the American Psychiatric Association.
** Numeric scale 1 to 100 that indicates the degree to which the clinical disorder has impaired patient's psychological, social and occupational functioning[2].

While making diagnosis or giving a pre-diagnostic 'impression' only, most clinician's listeners expect and wish to know for practical reasons:

- Is the patient depressed, maniacal or bipolar?
- Does the patient suffer from anxiety (which may be related to post-traumatic stress disorder; these patients are not psychotic!)?
- Is the patient psychotic?
- Is the patient demented?
- Is the patient delirious?
- Is the patient a substance abuser, intoxicated, or withdrawing?

- Does the patient adopt other risk behaviours?
- Does the patient have a personality disorder?
- Does the patient represent a risk to himself or herself (for example, self-mutilation)?
- Does his or her acute or chronic condition make him or her a threat to others and to whom?
- Is the patient dependent or independent socially?
- Does the patient risk breaking the law by antisocial behaviour, theft, rape, physical or mental aggression or abuse at home, at work, or in the community?

Many questions and assumptions about the case in both of the above-mentioned fields (medicine or surgery and psychiatry) are and should be evidence-based:

- Is the history information true and exact from a qualitative and quantitative point of view?
- How valid are the working diagnoses and diagnostic methods used?[1,3,4]
- How valid are the results of paraclinical tests given their external (reproducibility and representativity) and internal validity (sensibility, specificity, predictive values, etc.)?
- How much can an improvement after initial treatment be attributed to the medical or surgical treatment given?
- How efficient, effective, and efficacious is the treatment in similar cases and in cases of working and final diagnosis?
- What is the best evidence available from which to draw conclusions on the good or poor prognosis of a particular case?

4.1.2 Evidence-based clinical case reports

Answering such questions by searching and evaluating diagnostic, therapeutic or prognostic evidence, applied to the patient according to his or her general and clinical characteristics[4] is the foundation of an **evidence-based clinical case report.** Simply reporting clinical and paraclinical results, information and experience means taking them at face value, without questioning their validity and relevance to further decisions. In such cases, the ensuing patient management decisions are not always the most suitable.

An evidence-based case report can have two facets:

- In covering various components of a case report, such as diagnosis, treatment, or prognosis, a statement about them is accompanied by a powerful **'because ...'** explaining, on the basis of the best available evidence, the reason for the clinician's preferred option. The reasons for the conclusions drawn ('impression') should be clearly understandable.
- As in Reilly and Lemon's experience[5], the case **generates more general questions** to which answers are sought across the available evidence. The best possible solution to the patient's problem is then **applied back to** the question generating the **specific case**.

In this second instance, the evidence-based morning report takes on the following structure as proposed by Reilly and Lemon[5]. The example refers to Tandan *et al.*'s study[6] of colorectal carcinoma:

Components:	Example:
- **Patient identification**	
- **Admitting physician's identification**	
- **Clinical problem found in the patient** (N.B. Including a brief standard case report)	Patient recommended for admission and treatment for a metastatic colorectal cancer to the liver.
- **Search question**	Is the patient's long-term survival better after hepatic resection or hepatic cryosurgery?
- **Search answer**	Either intervention is worthy of consideration. However, most of the information available

	comes from case series reports. Controlled clinical trials have not been found. Valid conclusions cannot be made about the 5-year survival rate. Studies on hepatic resection show greater validity and consistency and survival rate of 20 per cent to 40 per cent.
• **Source of information**	Rapid Medline and Cancerlit search and Tandan et al.'s[6] critical review of the literature on this topic and question.
• **Quality of information**	Evidence is based mostly on case series studies; no controlled studies or trials were identified. The cryosurgery studies were methodologically poor, the resection studies were larger and more methodologically sound.
• **Potential impact on the care of my patient**	Although hepatic cryosurgery offers some unequivocal and other potential advantages over surgical hepatic resection, the evidence does not support its use in patients with resectable disease outside clinical trials. My patient should be preferably directed to the hepatic resection rather than to cryosurgery.

The purpose of this exercise is not to establish a general truth about a given problem, but rather to propose the best solution for a specific patient under care as seen in the more general evidence available.

How can we go once from raw clinical data in the form of an elementary observation to the clinical decision? Horton[7] proposes Toulmin's four-step evidence handling methodology:

- **Establish the warrant**, i.e. choose the justifiable: The patient has a tender abdominal wall (*défence musculaire*).
- **Clarify the backing**, i.e. determine how reliable the justifications are: A tender abdomen is almost always a sign of inflammation or bleeding.
- **Qualify the claim**, i.e. assess the magnitude of possible error and identify its sources: A board-like rigidity of the abdominal wall cannot be missed on physical examination if the physician is already familiar with the condition through past experiences. If present, there is a 10 per cent probability that the patient does not have an acute abdomen.
- **Define the conditions for rebuttal**, i.e. the elements that refute the claim. In this case, there are no systematic studies of a tender abdomen in cases where inflammation or bleeding is not involved.

Evidence-based conclusions about this case are the only goal of such EBM clinical case reporting. Clinical case reports of scientific value expand their discussion beyond the case.

However, even routine clinical cases can generate general questions that can subsequently be answered by an evidence-based approach. Should a particular diagnostic method be used? Should a conservative or radical treatment be considered a good choice in similar cases?[8]

The EBM practitioner should not become frustrated by the frequent lack of evidence and by the often seen lack of quality and completeness in this evidence. Here lies one of the challenges of medicine: to make the right decisions in situations of uncertainty and incomplete information and evidence. It is also the beauty of medicine and a huge reward for those who practise it correctly.

Clearly, different sources[1] (not just this book) must be used to learn, practice and teach EBM. Selected EBM principles and ways of thinking are presented here only as a way to correctly prepare, interpret and understand clinical case reports.

4.1.3 Discharge reports, notes and summaries

The discharge report focuses mainly on the post-admission evaluation of the case (diagnostic work-up), its course, management (treatment and care), prognosis at discharge, and orders and recommendations for further follow-up, treatment and care.

Discharge reports are valued for their succinct character and organization. For this reason, the clinician cannot discuss the full value of evidence used in a discharge summary. However, when full hospital data on the case are available, the clinician must be able to give, upon request, his or her opinion about the data's strength as evidence. How can the differential diagnosis process and its result be determined accurately? Does the response to the treatment support the general evidence in similar cases? Are the case's disease characteristics (extent, severity, stage) compatible with those of individuals who served as a source of prognostic studies and whose results are applied to this specific patient (case)?

Hence, discharge summaries must also be evidence-based.

4.2 CASE *AND* EVIDENCE PRESENTATIONS FOR CLAIMS IN OTHER SITUATIONS

Every problem related to health and disease is not solved behind the closed door of the hospital or doctor's office. Health issues are increasingly presented either to social bodies related to work and work environment, or at courts of law.

4.2.1 Case reports *with evidence* in occupational medicine

A clinical case is presented to the Worker Compensation Board or to another body for the purpose of obtaining some recognition of a health problem related to the occupational activity of the case. Most of these cases are routine.

The main challenge of the case presentation is not only to give a proper clinical picture of the problem in question, but also to relate it to the degree and frequency of exposure to the putative factor of a presumably occupational health problem, and to establish a prognosis in workable terms for all the decision makers involved (industry, law, etc.).

The demonstration of a cause–effect relationship must focus on some factor of interest related to the work and the workplace, as well as on the whole web of multiple causes in a given case. For example, while evaluating a case of chronic low back pain related to a static workload in forced protracted work positions, other possible causes of this health problem must be known and assessed, including if necessary: inflammatory and degenerative disorders of the musculoskeletal system, bone metastases, injury and post-traumatic consequences, neuropathies. The exclusion of competing hypotheses is paramount for all parties involved. Last but not least, the cause–effect relationship is crucial for patient treatment and follow-up.

Hence, the solidity of the clinical presentation of the case must be balanced with an equally structured and complete presentation of the exposure to putative factor(s) of the disease occurrence (risk) or its course (prognosis). This balance is certainly needed when respiratory problems in the workplace are involved.

Risk or prognostic factors may be of a physical, chemical, biological, social, or psychological nature. Their frequency and intensity should be made clear. For how long was the subject exposed to toxic fumes? What was the frequency and intensity to concentration spikes (episodes) of exposure? Have there been any quantitative or qualitative individual (masks) and/or collective (ventilation) countermeasures? Were there other putative factors such as smoking creating a network of causes for the clinical problem under consideration?

The cause–effect relationship must be evaluated in view of a general knowledge of this problem. How strong is the evidence that a particular toxic fume causes a given respiratory problem? How specific is it? How does it respond to other criteria of causality[9]?

A case with unknown aetiology will rely on a demonstration of **analogy** (similar circumstances or conditions, other diseases of better known aetiology). However, analogy is only one of several causal criteria, as defined today[9].

An important question arises: **Does general evidence apply to the case presented for compensation?**

Usually, the case presented for compensation is admissible depending on the demographic and clinical characteristics of the groups taking part in clinical trials or aetiological observational studies and that have demonstrated a somewhat causal link between a presumably putative factor and the disease under study. Does the patient belong to the same target group? Even better: is he/she comparable to other exposed individuals who developed a similar health problem? And how is he/she comparable to the unexposed individuals who have developed the health problem anyway? Are proofs based on original studies only or are they based on a systematic review of evidence (meta-analysis)? What is the quality of such evidence?

Knowledge of clinical and field epidemiology, meta-analysis and systematic review of evidence are necessary to relate general knowledge to the case.

The onus of providing proof is on the requester and his or her physician.

In view of the above-mentioned considerations, we can understand the architecture of a case report in occupational medicine as reworked from Hall[10]:

Purpose of the report	Questions and expectations for which this report should provide answers.
Past history	Focus on pre-existing problems and their management relevant to the present case.

Current situation	Focus mainly on the patient's past and current integration or reintegration in his or her work environment and status.
Summary standard clinical case report	Highlight topics, data, and information relevant to the presented case.
Conclusion	Answers to questions and expectations raised at the beginning of the report.
	Proper distinctions are made between the disorder (intrinsic situation), impairment (exteriorized), disability (objectified), and handicap (socialized).
	Current need and plans for treatment, rehabilitation, occupational reintegration or change, social support, and follow-up.
	Conclusions about questioned and questionable causal and prognostic factors.

In this context, it should not be forgotten that occupational and environmental data and information from research supporting the presentation and interpretation of an occupational clinical case are of unequal quality[11].

4.2.2 Case reports *with evidence* in tort litigations

Clinical cases are often heard in the Courts. Usually, a party subject to the occurrence of physical or mental harm presents its presumed cause along with a request for compensation.

To solve problems under litigation, physicians and lawyers from one continent or country to another may use different ways of thinking about causes and their effect. **Health scientists** are replacing positivism–corpuscularianism which originated in the 19th century by a combination of deductive and inductive reasoning and by probabilistic thinking. **Lawyers, judges and juries**, as Brennan[12] points out, tend to assume the existence of a clearly delineated causal chain. They try to identify a *'but for* cause', i.e. the event that, but for its existence, another event would not have occurred. Given a possible multifactorial aetiology or web of causes of a health problem, courts also use the notion of *proximate cause*, i.e. policies that the judge wishes to reinforce in his finding of liability.

The paradigm of causation in law often bears a close resemblance to *corpuscularianism*, i.e. characterizing causation as collisions that follow the physical laws defined by mathematics[12]. However, law increasingly accepts the deductive and probabilistic reasoning and argumentation by health professionals.

In toxic tort litigations, toxicological evidence relies on four sources; structure-activity relationships, short-term molecular screening tests, animal bioassays and epidemiological studies. To prevent courts slipping into corpuscularian habits and accepting untested anecdotal theories, physicians are expected to identify the source of evidence on which they rely, how that evidence relates to the other evidence available[12], and last but not least, **how the evidence applies specifically to the case** (patient), plaintiff in the face of law. All these tasks are not easy.

4.2.2.1 Civil versus criminal cases

In **civil courts**, the following types of event are frequent: a father is injured in a traffic accident and his insurance agency claims compensation from another party who supposedly caused the accident in question; a few office employees launch a class action suit claiming that their work environment causes them to have cancer; the tobacco industry is brought to trial and held responsible for respiratory and cardiovascular problems, distressing long-term users of their product. Guilt must be shown to be **more probable than improbable, without any reasonable doubt**.

In **criminal courts**, when a child dies as a result of family abuse, a suspect parent's role must be demonstrated **without any doubt**: '. . . it could not happen otherwise . . .'

A properly worked-up clinical case report and **evidence** are presented here. The demonstration of a possible cause–effect relationship is the responsibility of the plaintiff and precedes an effort to disprove it by the defence. The clinical case reporters for the plaintiff must know that. They must go well beyond the description of the case and their clinical skill in case reporting should be matched by:

- an evaluation of the solidity of the general evidence; and by
- the demonstration that such evidence applies to the case presented to the court.

The latter is usually the greatest challenge. In general, the court's role is to make decisions about the case of the plaintiff and not about an identical problem beyond the case.

As in occupational health, a clinical case presented in court describes in considerable detail the patient's history and the quantity, duration and frequency of peak exposure to presumed physical, chemical or biological aetiological factors. Clinical experience in case presentations is matched by the definition and quantification of the cause. Also, the case rests and is supported by an assessment of putative factors on the basis of general evidence provided by evidence-based public health and medicine.

A good description of the case must be matched by an equally good analysis and explanation of this event. Today, the professional and scientific quality and objectivity of the case is considered an integral part of medical ethics. Falsification, hiding or distortion of facts and evidence are unethical.

4.2.2.2 Beyond a simple case description. Demonstration of the role of a factor presumed responsible

In epidemiology, a suspected cause–effect relationship such as smoking and lung cancer is evaluated based on either: assumptions from observational descriptive and analytical (aetiologic) research, experimental proof, or both of the above.

The criteria of a cause–effect relationship are increasingly numerous and more structured[9]. They include:

- **prerequisites**, such as exclusion of chance, consistency with prediction, logical building of studies, clinimetrically valid data, unbiased observations, comparisons and analysis and avoidance of uncontrollable and uninterpretable factors in studies;
- **major criteria**, such as temporality, strength, manifestational and causal specificity, biological gradient, consistency and biological plausibility;
- **conditional criteria**, such as coherence with prevalent knowledge and analogy;
- **experimental proof as a reference criterion.**

Health professionals usually refer to these criteria when evaluating evidence found in the literature or in their own research. In court, they must place the criteria within the context of 'daily life'.

Solidity of evidence does not depend on the authority of the presenter or of any other actor in a court case. It must be built from scratch in the court itself. This allows the court to be free and independent from a prevalent general feeling about the problem, which may not be necessarily right.

Three major criteria of causality are routinely quantified in epidemiology[9]:

- The **strength** of an association in terms of a **relative risk**.
- The **specificity** of an association estimated among others according to the importance of an **attributable risk** and **aetiological fraction**.
- The **biological gradient** of all the above.

When studying relative risk, an occurrence of an event (usually disease incidence in studies of risk, or case fatality rate in studies of prognosis) is compared as a ratio between individuals exposed and those unexposed to a putative factor. The higher the value of the relative risk, the stronger the association is going to be.

While studying how specific or exclusive the disease occurrence or course is in relation to the factor of interest, an important difference is determined between rates in exposed and unexposed individuals (attributable risk), i.e. the proportion of an entire risk in exposed individuals due to the factor under study among all other possible factors representing a network of causes of a health problem (aetiological fraction, attributable risk percent).

If only one causal factor is known, an attributable (aetiological) fraction higher than 50 per cent suggests that an event is more probable than improbable if exposed to the putative factor. If more than one causal factor is known, the aetiological fraction, attributable to the factor of interest should be more important than any other competing factor, or better, superior to all other factors put together.

However, purely quantitative epidemiological thinking must be paired with the assessment of biological, clinical and social plausibility, and other considerations specific to the problem under court evaluation.

Finally, the ultimate challenge may be to **demonstrate that general knowledge applies to the clinical case presented in court**. At the very least, the clinical case presenter is required to show that demographic (age, sex, occupation, etc.), clinical (disease stage, prognosis, treatment, etc.) and other relevant characteristics of the patient (case) are compatible with similar characteristics present in individuals on which 'general' research was done. As statisticians ask: 'Would this person be eligible to enter the aetiologic study or trial and does this person come from the same population as the individuals representing the research group?'

In other situations, the court looks at the **precedents**. Have similar or analogous cases been handled by the courts in the past and what was the verdict at that time? Any discrepancy with respect to the previous cases is usually held against the case in question.

Today, health professionals and lawyers are working together on building a common logic, philosophy, and understanding of cause–effect relationships, which interest medicine and law as well[13]. From a larger body of literature[14-19], only some of the most important principles were outlined here. It is increasingly expected that a clinical case reporter in court understand such common thinking and the language of medicine and law while presenting 'his/her' case (patient) as a jurist and practitioner of law.

4.3 CONCLUSIONS

Even routine clinical case reports related to any scientific discovery require a clear focus and organization. Moreover, they are increasingly presented with a critical appraisal and interpretation of evidence of its causal factors, therapeutic success, and effectiveness of preventive measures or prognosis.

Physicians strive to master the following:

- Conveying communication (listening and talking to the patient).
- Assessing patient risks.
- Making diagnosis and prognosis.
- Problem listing and hierarchical classification.
- Decision making (making choices).
- Performance (mastery of exploratory or surgical procedures).
- Management of the patient after intervention (follow-up and care, control of disease course).
- Evaluation of the effectiveness and efficiency of cure and care.
- Respect of medical, cultural and social ethics as well as patient's values, preferences, and expectations.
- Empathy.

Even an 'ordinary' clinical case report should reflect these virtues since:

- A case involves a continuous search, evaluation, and use of evidence in decisions, interpretation of findings, and outlining of further steps of patient (case) management.
- From a methodological point of view, any case report, routine or 'scientific' is at a halfway point between the 'hard' practice of clinimetrics and the 'soft' practice of qualitative research.

If we look at the sequence of steps in clinical practice that follow the case from its history through the observation, interpretation, diagnosis, treatment, and prognosis to outcomes[9], only the proportion of qualitative and quantitative methodology changes. The qualitative component is more prevalent at the beginning of the pre-clinical and clinical course of the case. The quantitative component takes over gradually towards the final outcome in the patient.

Greenhalgh's **narrative-based medicine**[20] concept focuses mainly on the better qualitative information provided by the patient and used in subsequent clinical decision making.

If the quality of clinical data and information is to improve:

- Clinical epidemiologists must be familiar with the **methodology of qualitative research**[21], know how to use it and how to discover independent and dependent variables of interest for quantitative research either from experience, from past quantitative research, or from past or present qualitative research.
- Qualitative research practitioners must master particularly **clinimetrics**[21,9] from the whole body of clinical epidemiology. This will help them to use the clear clinimetric criteria necessary for any observation in medical setting.

The results of such an amalgam should be promising. However, if the idea of doing some research in the qualitative field[22] applied to clinical case reporting sounds appealing, beware! At present, research grant providers strongly prefer quantitative explorations!

We have just barely begun to establish the 'rules' of such an evidence-based approach and to gather the required experience. A flexible evidence approach, wherever possible and relevant, is definitely a better alternative than a simple educated guess. However, the former will never entirely replace the latter.

What else should a 'scientific' clinical case report include? The answer is discussed in the following chapter.

REFERENCES

1. Sackett DL, Richardson SW, Rosenberg W, Haynes RB. *Evidence-based Medicine. How to Practice and Teach EBM*. New York: Churchill Livingstone, 1977.
2. Carlat D. *The Psychiatric Interview. A Practical Guide*. Philadelphia: Lippincott Williams & Wilkins, 1999.
3. Sackett DL. A primer on precision and accuracy of the clinical examination. *JAMA*, 1992; **267**: 2638–44.
4. Hatala R, Smieja M, Kane S-L, Cook DJ, Meade MO, Nishikawa J. An evidence-based approach to the clinical examination. *J Gen Intern Med, (JGIM)*, 1997; **12**: 182–7.
5. Reilly B, Lemon M. Evidence-based morning report: A popular new format in a large teaching hospital. *Am J Med*, 1997; **103**: 419–26.

6. Tandan VR, Harmantas A, Gallinger S. Long-term survival after hepatic cryosurgery versus surgical resection for metastatic colorectal carcinoma: a critical review of the literature. *Can J Surg*, 1997; **40**: 175–81.

7. Horton R. The grammar of interpretive medicine. *CMAJ*, 1998; **159**: 245–9.

8. Towards evidence based emergency medicine: best BETS from Manchester Royal Infirmary. Edited by K Mackway-Jones. *J Accid Emerg Med*, 1999; **16**: 362–6.

9. Jenicek M. *Epidemiology. The Logic of Modern Medicine*. Montreal: EPIMED International, 1995. (See Section 6.3: Fundamental philosophy and criteria of the cause-effect relationship. pp. 162–8.)

10. Hall MC. *Independent Medical Examination for Insurance and Legal Reports*. Toronto and Vancouver: Butterworths, 1998.

11. Rushton L. Reporting of occupational and environmental research: use and misuse of statistical and epidemiological methods. *Occup Environ Med*, 2000; **57**:1–9.

12. Brennan TA. Untangling causation issues in law and medicine: Hazardous substance litigation. *Ann Intern Med*, 1987; **107**: 741–7.

13. Epidemiologic proof of causality in court. Physician's contribution to decisions in tort litigations. pp. 192–4 in: Jenicek M. *Epidemiology. The Logic of Modern Medicine*. Montreal: EPIMED International, 1995.

14. Black B, Lilienfeld DE. Epidemiologic proof in toxic tort litigation. *Fordham Law Review*, 1984; **52**: 732–85.

15. Brennan TA, Carter RF. Legal and scientific probability of causation of cancer and other environmental disease in individuals. *J Health Politics Law*, 1985; **10**: 33–80.

16. Lilienfeld DE, Black B. The epidemiologist in court: some comments. *Am J Epidemiol*, 1986; **123**: 961–4.

17. Teret SP. Litigating for the public's health. *AJPH*, 1986; **76**: 1027–9.

18. Cole P. Epidemiologist as an expert witness. *J Clin Epidemiol*, 1991; **44**(Suppl 1): 35S-39S.

19. Holden C. Science in court. *Science*, 1989; **243**: 1658–9.

20. Greenhalgh T. Narrative based medicine in an evidence based world. *BMJ*, 1999; **318**: 323–5.

21. Feinstein AR. *Clinimetrics*. New Haven and London: Yale University Press, 1987.

22. Silverman D. *Doing Qualitative Research. A Practical Handbook*. London: SAGE Publications, 2000.

CHAPTER 5

How to prepare
a single case
report: from a
literary essay to
the report of
evidence

How many times have we heard our senior colleagues declare: 'since he can't do clinical research, let him report clinical cases'? Yet the case study is an important and integral part of clinical research. It is our duty to grant it its own letters of nobility, by providing it with a logic, a methodology, an architecture and a series of objectives comparable in their rigour to those of other types of research in medicine: aetiological research, evaluation of diagnostic methods, clinical trials, and studies of prognosis.

CHAPTER 5

How to prepare a single case report: from a literary essay to the report of evidence

A clinical case report is a form of verbal or written communication with its own specific rules, that is produced for professional and scientific purposes. It usually focuses on an unusual single event (patient or

clinical situation) in order to provide a better understanding of the case and of its effects on improved
clinical decision-making.

In their instructions to contributors, medical journals generally
specify the required length of text (number of words) and newness
of observation and nothing more. However, there are many other
guidelines to follow.

The study and reporting of cases in clinical practice occurs at
two different levels, as outlined below.

1. **Routine case reports** (admissions and discharges) ensure the
    continuity of ward activities or outline those activities directly
    related to the proper functioning of the hospital.
2. **Case reports of scientific value**, usually topics of grand rounds
    and reports in medical journals, focus on:
    - case reports;
    - case reports with a literature review;
    - case series reports;
    - systematic reviews of cases.

This second category presents the most challenges.

There are common rules for all the above-mentioned categories
of clinical case reports. Both general explanations of these rules and
specific recommendations will follow in this text, which focuses
mainly on clinical case reports of scientific value.

Do we really need to investigate this area? Should we not be
satisfied with the existing literature?

In reality, the bibliographic heritage of medical casuistics is not
very rich, especially that pertaining to case reporting methodology.
Aside from clinical epidemiological investigations of case reports,
the past 20 years have generally only produced 'how to' articles
covering either routine ward case reporting[1-4], the content[5-8] and
form[9-12] of the case report, or strategies to adopt in order to ensure
the case report's publication[13,14].

More recently, however, editors have begun to state their expectations more precisely[5,15-17], although some of these expectations
differ from the supporting literature and some aren't backed up by

the available methodology in the medical press. In this chapter, we will attempt to create a stronger bond between the content and the form of the product in order to meet consumer expectations.

As already mentioned, clinical case reports must be seen as the first link in the chain of evidence. Reliance on clinical epidemiology, clinimetrics and an evidence-based approach to medical information requires additional considerations. How, without epidemiology, can a case reporter qualify the risk and prognostic characteristics of his case? How, without clinimetrics, can the clinical and paraclinical features of a case be presented in operational and measurable terms? How can the evidence (weak or not) that emerges from a case be compared with other evidence from fields related to the case?

The case report must be as solid as a rock or as the other pieces of evidence associated with the problem under study.

5.1 ROUTINE WARD CASE REPORTS AND HOSPITAL-FOCUSED CASE PRESENTATIONS

Routine case reports are the most ubiquitous of all single case reports. Rather than a verbatim retelling of the admission work-up, they should represent a 'medical reporting'[1], a succinct account of an event.

Such case presentations, repeated in time, usually follow an expanded 'SOAP' structure[3], which should be more than familiar to any North American house staff member preparing daily progress notes on his patients:

- Presenting the problem.
- Subjective history of present illness, and personal and family history.
- Objective data (clinical and paraclinical, course so far).
- Assessment (diagnosis, differential diagnosis, co-morbidity review).
- Plans of treatment and care, including their evaluation in terms of material and human resources (management of the case).
- Discussion.

In psychiatry, important additions are made, as reviewed in Chapter 4.

We should note that a case work-up and report are not only the result of a properly conducted interview[4,18] (including review of systems), but also a structured synthesis of additional elements such as paraclinical work-ups and results, outcome assessments and social evaluations (e.g. reintegration into the patient's family, professional and social environment).

A much greater challenge is presented when cases are reported for the advancement of knowledge and science.

5.2 CLINICAL CASE REPORTING AS A SCIENTIFIC CONTRIBUTION TO EVIDENCE IN MEDICINE

Let us stress again that a clinical case report is a form of scientific and professional communication. As such, it has its own rules. Surprisingly, most medical journals give prospective authors no indications other than those related to the newness of the topic and the volume of the text (number of words). More details are clearly needed.

The success of a clinical case report depends on four major criteria:

- the relevance of the topic;
- the value of the presentation (precision, organization, structure);
- the knowledge that this case contributes to the existing general information about the topic;
- the clarity of the elements that can be retained for practice, research, or both.

Hence, a good clinical case report must:

- be written according to the preset requirements;

- contain all essential elements, in a complete and well-structured manner;
- convey an unambiguous message.

Readers who believe that they do not need clinical epidemiology and biostatistics to present a single case, may have to think again. Even a particular case should be analysed in the context of the pathology it represents and in the framework of a particular clinical practice. In one way or another, the case should be compared with what is considered usual and general.

5.2.1 Single case reports

Single case reports fall into several categories:

- Either a *'classical case report'* is produced, where all necessary components and the discussion are limited to the case and the problem it represents, or
- a case is presented as a *'brief report'* in journals such as *The Lancet,* with only the most essential elements published (four typed pages or a half-page printed), or
- *'a case to learn from'* is prepared. The *New England Journal of Medicine* has created two sections for this type of case. In the Clinical Problem Solving section, the case is presented step by step by a seasoned clinician. The author shares with the reader the experience of going from one stage of the report to another. In the Case Records of the Massachusetts General Hospital Weekly Clinicopathological Exercises, the case is presented in its entirety. A pathologist then re-evaluates it.

5.2.2 Requirements and expectations regarding clinical case reports

Any successful clinical case reporter must keep in mind several considerations, desirable attributes and necessary components of a good report before sitting down to prepare it. The following suggestions are a reflection of the requirements and expectations laid out by medical journals for a good case report[15–17]. They should increase the author's chance of being published. The saying that your sleep will be only as good as the way you make your bed is valid here as well.

All case reports must be prepared with a specific reason in mind and must be based on high quality clinical data.

5.2.2.1 Reasons and motives for a clinical case report

When the time of year for promotions arrives, many clinicians feel a sudden urge to report clinical cases in order to enhance their list of publications. However, there are nineteen more serious reasons to publish a case report (see Table 5.1). These reasons should be stated in the introduction of all clinical case reports and, ideally, any one of these reasons should help to refocus clinical decisions.

However, everything depends on the relevance of the case. Riesenberg[18] notes that, from a recent selection of fifty-one land-

Table 5.1 – Reasons and motives for a case report

1. Unusual presentation of unknown aetiology.
2. Unusual natural history.
3. Unusual natural or clinical courses (spectrum, gradient, prognosis).
4. Challenging differential diagnosis.
5. Mistake in diagnosis, its causes and consequences.
6. Unusual and/or unexpected effect of treatment.
7. Diagnostic and therapeutic 'accidents' (causes, consequences, remedies).
8. Unusual co-morbidity (its diagnosis, treatment, outcome).
9. Transfer of medical technology (disease, organ, system).
10. Unusual setting of medical care.
11. Management of an emergency case.
12. Patient compliance.
13. Patient/doctor interaction (as in psychiatry).
14. Single case clinical trial ('n-of-1' study).
15. Clinical situation which cannot be reproduced for ethical reasons.
16. Limited access to cases.
17. New medical technology (use, outcomes, consequences).
18. Confirmation of something already known (only if useful for a 'systematic case report review and synthesis').
19. Solving a challenging problem in medical ethics.

mark articles in medicine[19], five are *'just a simple'* case report. For example, Levine and Stetson published 'An unusual case of intra-group agglutination'[20]. This careful observation of one single case led the authors to conclude[21] that the majority of cases of erythro-blastosis fetalis resulted from isoimmunization of an Rh-negative mother by the Rh-positive red blood cells of the fetus. Greenwalt mentions that *'some may scoff at the publication of case reports, but for the astute scientist, a carefully documented study of an unusual patient represents an experiment of nature that may be the opportunity to explain a long-recorded but unexplained clinical mystery. Some credit must also go to the editorial staff of The Journal for having pub-lished this'*[22].

Sometimes, the message of the case report is missed because the reader does not know the desirable attributes of a good clinical case report, how to interpret a case report, and where extrapolations, generalizations and applications of a report should stop. All efforts made by the authors and the publishing journal would be futile in this situation.

5.2.2.2 Selection and quality of the clinical and paraclinical data on which a report is based

Selection of data

It is impossible to reproduce everything that a clinician has seen. Editorial space is limited.

The objective of the case report is not to prove that the clinician has done his job properly but rather to offer all information neces-sary for the understanding of the problem illustrated by the case. A 'classical' casuist searches for and provides all in-depth details of the case. A clinical casuist 'goes for the jugular' by providing just the essential information[23].

Data should be provided to allow the reader to understand the other steps of the case reporter's work, the differential diagnosis, or the choice of the treatment. A case report on a complicated excision of a cyst in an unusual and surgically challenging part of the inguinal region does not necessarily require an explanation of the patient's normal chest X-ray or glycaemia.

Quality of data

Quality of data counts even if it is not evident in a brief report itself.

A case report provides *clinical data* (for example, that a patient's blood pressure is 180/110mmHg) as well as *clinical information* (the fact that the patient suffers from hypertension) as an interpretation of raw observations (data).

The reporter must have at hand and be ready to explain, on request, his measurement techniques and his inclusion and exclusion criteria for given information, readings or recording in *operational* terms. *Conceptual* criteria are not enough.

Soft data such as nausea, pain, anxiety, loneliness, puffiness and swelling, so well known to family doctors or psychiatrists, represent a special challenge. Their definitions should be as close as possible to those of **hard data**. Hard data come largely from the paraclinical (laboratory) area: blood count, urinary output, ventricular ejection fraction etc. Methods for *hardening of soft data* are discussed in the current epidemiological literature[24-26]. For example, measurement of the severity of pain may be attempted using an appropriate scale, or a degree of confusion in an elderly patient may be evaluated by an *ad hoc* psychiatric questionnaire.

A clinical case reporter should keep a record of his data collection and interpretation, in order to offer adequate explanations, should the need arise.

A well-presented case based on valid data follows the same rules as any other research topic would[27].

5.2.2.3 Content and structure of a single case report

A journal's space and requirements permitting, a clinical case report should have five distinct sections (see Table 5.2).

Title

Two kinds of titles are found in the literature. The first are symbolic or poetic titles, some of which possess advertising qualities. For example, a title like 'The rooster that sang a different song' as an introduction to a case report on an unusual clinical picture of whooping cough may perhaps reflect the author's wit and draw attention. However, the reader might have to read through the whole report in order to understand what it is about. If, as in

Table 5.2 – The five sections of a clinical case report

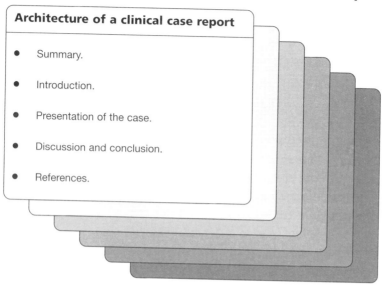

Architecture of a clinical case report
• Summary.
• Introduction.
• Presentation of the case.
• Discussion and conclusion.
• References.

Agatha Christie's or Sir Arthur Conan Doyle's novels, the mystery is unravelled only at the end of the clinical case report, its reading is often painful. Usually this type of structure suggests that the author wanted to say: 'look how clever I am'.

The other kind of title is one that directly informs the readers about the problem and the topic. It conveys the elements of a well-formulated research question. In original research or in systematic reviews, research questions should reflect the following train of thoughts:

intervention → **outcomes** →
population setting and **condition of interest**[28].

For example[28]:

'Does **anticoagulation therapy** improve **outcomes** in **patients** with **ischaemic stroke?**'

or[29]:

'Do **anticoagulant agents** improve **outcomes** in **patients with acute ischaemic stroke** compared with **no treatment?**'

Similar principles apply to titles of case reports. The informative title (or research question) is definitely preferable for a clinical case report. For example, the case report that is analysed and annotated in the next chapter is entitled '**Electrocardiographic changes** suggestive of **cardiac ischaemia** in a **patient** with **oesophageal food impaction**'[30]. The reader immediately knows the diagnostic intervention of interest (ECG), its outcome (changes suggestive of cardiac ischaemia), the population and the condition of interest (patient with oesophageal food impaction). He may decide if this topic interests him and whether he wants to read the rest. Only the subtitle is symbolic and allegorical, since it acts as an attention grabber: 'A case that's hard to swallow'. It should be noted that if the subtitle had been the main title, an uninformed reader might not have known what to expect. In other words, the title should always get right to the point.

Summary

A summary of any professional communication has two objectives:

- to attract the reader to the topic in a striking and organized manner; and
- to convey the most important highlights to a busy reader.

Many high impact journals including *The Lancet, JAMA, The New England Journal of Medicine* and *Annals of Internal Medicine* require well-structured summaries[31-33] for medical research articles. Independent of the nature of the article, a summary should give some background information about the problem, while also stating the objective, the design, the setting, the subjects, the results of the study and their meaning. Table 5.3 shows that a similar structure applies to the summary of a clinical case report.

For example, summaries constructed as above are expected to introduce clinical case reports in special Case Reports issues of the *Obstetrics and Gynecology* and *Revue de Pédiatrie* journals.

Introduction

In this section, the case has to be 'sold' to the reader, especially if there is no summary. It should persuade him or her to read through the whole text. It should also give all the necessary information about the problem under study.

Four kinds of information should be included in the introduction. Table 5.4 summarizes them.

Table 5.3 – Organization of the summary

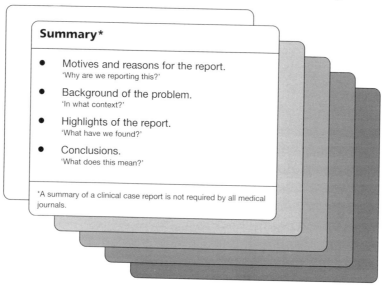

Summary*

- Motives and reasons for the report.
  'Why are we reporting this?'

- Background of the problem.
  'In what context?'

- Highlights of the report.
  'What have we found?'

- Conclusions.
  'What does this mean?'

*A summary of a clinical case report is not required by all medical journals.

Table 5.4 – Organization of the introduction

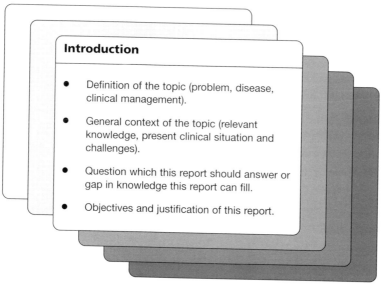

Introduction

- Definition of the topic (problem, disease, clinical management).

- General context of the topic (relevant knowledge, present clinical situation and challenges).

- Question which this report should answer or gap in knowledge this report can fill.

- Objectives and justification of this report.

Let us now examine in greater detail some components of the introduction.

Problem under study. The topic of a case report can be new[5,23,34,35] for the reasons already summarized in Table 5.1. Therefore, the value of the case report would depend partly on the documentation of the newness of the concepts advanced by the case or on the possible resulting modifications[36,37] of the currently accepted view of the problem.

The newness of a case report may be categorized in three ways:

1. A very ordinary situation may present unusual features or occur in an unusual setting. For example, *Salmonella typhi* osteomyelitis of the sternum was noted in an immunocompetent patient[38]. Elsewhere, *Salmonella* skull osteomyelitis was observed[39].
2. A rare or forgotten disease whose typical features have appeared in recent times in a specific setting (e.g. necrotizing fasciitis), thus leading to the improvement of diagnostic and timely treatment techniques.
3. Sometimes, although a certain disease has supposedly been eradicated, a few case reports in the literature can be indicative of a new occurrence (endemicity, pandemic or epidemic).

Background and general context of the problem. A very succinct review of the problem tells the author whether or not a case[5] should be reported. An adequate literature search is also necessary for the author to know what clinical and paraclinical data should be gathered and studied.

Origins and motives of the report. Does the question under study relate to the risk assessment, diagnosis, treatment or prognosis? Does it lead to a better choice from a set of possible clinical decisions? A reader with less clinical experience will especially benefit from such explicit information.

Objectives and justification of the report. Specifying the expected results with regard to practice and/or research is probably the most difficult part of stating the relevance of the report. Despite this, the report's justification should always be present, either in this section or in the conclusion of the case report (with the addition made by the contribution to our knowledge of the problem).

Presentation of the case

This section is the core of the message. Table 5.5 summarizes its components.

A clinical case report is an exercise in **clinimetrics**[25,26], originally defined as *the measurement of clinical data*[25], or as *the field concerned with indexes, rating scales and other expressions used to describe or measure symptoms, physical signs or other distinctly clinical phenomena in clinical medicine*[40,41] *in view of clinical decision making*[26]. It is also an exercise in **hermeneutics**, i.e. in *interpretation and understanding*[42]. Now, the reader may be wondering: 'Do I do really need all this?'. The answer is, definitely. Although this process occurs most often unconsciously, it may also take place consciously in accordance with a certain structure.

Table 5.5 – Components of the section presenting the case

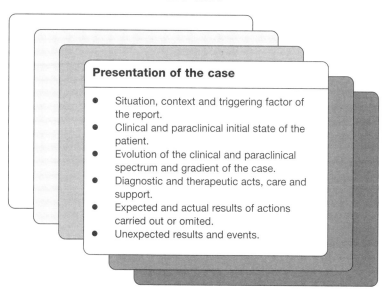

Presentation of the case

- Situation, context and triggering factor of the report.
- Clinical and paraclinical initial state of the patient.
- Evolution of the clinical and paraclinical spectrum and gradient of the case.
- Diagnostic and therapeutic acts, care and support.
- Expected and actual results of actions carried out or omited.
- Unexpected results and events.

Thinking and evaluation in clinical epidemiology are based on the paradigm of a simple sequence: **initial state → action (manoeuvre) → subsequent state**[24,26,43] that is often tricky to apply, analyse and interpret in many actual situations. Clinical case presentations follow a pattern similar to the one illustrated in Figure 5.1.

1. **Antecedents and development of the case**. This includes family and personal history, exposure to aetiologic factors and incubation periods plus developments of the disease in its induction period.
2. The **initial state** is the moment at which the case report begins.
3. Clinical and paraclinical **manoeuvres** or **actions** follow. They may be diagnostic in nature such as serum ferritin measurement, magnetic resonance examination, neurological assessment etc. The probability of diagnosis before and after results (initial and subsequent state) is also reviewed. This may involve drug treatment or surgery with the expectation of a better subsequent state.
4. The **subsequent state** or **result (outcome)** is then outlined, i.e. better health, a cure, unexpected complications, adverse effects.
5. Finally, ensuing **clinical decisions** are presented with regards to the treatment, the improvement and expansion of the diagnostic work-up, and the precautions to be taken in similar cases and situations.

A case report should always contain these steps in an easy to understand format.

The management of every case should follow the chronological sequence illustrated in Figure 5.2, with its alternate data collection, diagnostic process, treatment and effect and patient outcomes. One or several feedback loops within this cascading structure are common. A case report should also allow the reader to understand the steps that the author took to progress through such a sequence.

CLINICAL CASE REPORTING

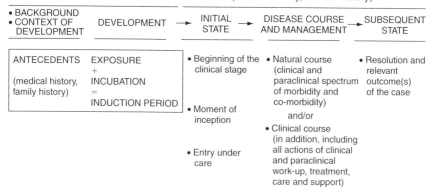

Figure 5.1 – Stages of the case

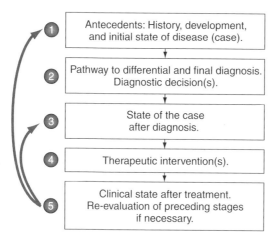

Figure 5.2 – Sequence of case management

Existing situation in the field of interest and triggering factor of the report. The reader of a case report is not necessarily as familiar with the pathology and its clinical management as the author. A summary of current practices and acquired experience generally accepted in the field should be presented. The reason for the report should also be given.

For example, the challenges and highlights of a particular cancer treatment should be related first. Then, the unexpected adverse effects of treatment should be outlined (nausea, abnormal neurological, haematological and biochemical findings, haemorrhagic enterocolitis, anaphylactoid reactions etc.). The author of the report should then explain which expensive intensive care and critical outcomes in the patient should be avoided in the future, if a subsequent pharmaco-epidemiological study showed a cause–effect relationship between the treatment and its suspected undesirable effects, as suggested by the reported case.

Initial clinical and paraclinical state of the patient. Often, clinical data (interview, bedside examination and follow-up) and paraclinical data (microbiology, haematology, biochemistry, imaging techniques etc.) should be identified according to their role in the study and management of the pathology in question.

Patient characteristics. From a patient's history and physical examination, several *risk characteristics* can be identified. It should be specified which of these are *risk factors* (modifiable, such as smoking, physical inactivity or eating habits) and which are *risk markers* (non-modifiable, such as age, sex or race). Risk characteristics precede the onset of the disease, just as smoking precedes lung cancer. Other characteristics still present or appearing after the onset of disease are of equal interest as *prognostic characteristics*, sometimes modifiable (*prognostic factors*), sometimes not (*prognostic markers*). Certain readers consider these subtleties truly important for decision making. From such 'networks of risk or prognostic characteristics' causal associations may be hypothesized or quantified if their strength and specificity are known. Further details belong to the field of epidemiology[26].

Course of the disease. As a result of drawing a picture based on direct experience and patient charts, less experienced reporters tend to provide all details from a clinical and paraclinical follow-up in order to assure their peers and case report recipients that nothing was forgotten and that the work-up and follow-up were complete.

Only essential information for case understanding is necessary. By way of example, why should normal levels of uric acid in body fluids in an overwhelming and fast evolving necrotizing fasciitis be reported if this information is not essential for decision making?

Nevertheless, some protocol of case reporting will be required sooner or later, even if it is only going to be kept at hand. It is also useful if readers raise additional questions about the management of the case: How was the normality of an observation defined in operational terms? If an outlying observation was made, was it a statistical outlier, or was it a clinical outlier implying different medical or surgical management? Was it an abnormality in terms of appearance, localization, tissue composition, function, rhythm, frequency, direction, volume, speed etc.?

Were the exploratory surgical procedure (e.g. access of a fibreoptic catheter) and the surgery itself (e.g. laparoscopic cholecystectomy) normal?

Evolution of the case's clinical spectrum and gradient.   It is not always easy to describe a clinical course. Challenges lie in the identification of the beginning stages of the case and of the disease occurrence, in the follow-up of the disease spectrum and gradient, in the study of the co-morbidity, and in knowing where to stop.

Beginning of the case.   This point in time is sometimes quite difficult to determine. The period of exposure often overlaps or blends with the incubation period of the case. Smoking and chronic obstructive lung disease is an example of this. The starting point of the disease may be insidious and the first mild spells might go unnoticed. The disease does not necessarily begin at the moment when the physician sees his patient for the first time. The problem of exposure and incubation is somehow obviated by epidemiologists who consider the sum of both these periods as an *induction period of the disease.*

Disease spells.   Is the first reported spell of a disease really the first? This is not simply an academic question. If the spell is really the first, the situation is one of disease incidence. Related characteristics are then interpreted as *risk factors.* Any subsequent spell is considered an expression of the *point prevalence* of the health problem and the related characteristics are interpreted as *prognostic factors.* Ensuing clinical decisions are quite different. Smoking is a powerful risk factor for lung cancer, but no one has yet demonstrated convincingly that stopping smoking after the diagnosis of lung cancer meaningfully improves the patient's prognosis.

Angina, epilepsy, migraine, arthritis, amyotrophic lateral sclerosis, Alzheimer's and Parkinson's disease all fall into the challenging category of clinimetrics and epidemiological interpretation of findings.

Needless to say, all spells should be observed and measured equally well in terms of their timing, duration and amplitude. Remissions that distinguish them from another should also be studied.

Cases as part of the clinical spectrum. The clinical spectrum, like the colour spectrum, primarily reflects the variability of the clinical picture and the extent of the disease. For example, the ocular, ulceroglandular or respiratory manifestations of tularaemia indicate that this disease has an extended clinical spectrum. The common cold, however, has a very limited clinical spectrum.

In many clinical reports, greater attention is paid to the paraclinical spectrum. Nevertheless, it should be noted that the clinical spectrum of signs and symptoms merits equal attention and a rigorously structured description.

Cases as part of the clinical gradient. Studying the gradient of a disease is synonymous with studying its severity. Non-apparent cases, flu-like cases, symptomatic hepatitis and fulminant hepatitis reflect an extended gradient of viral hepatitis. Again, the clinical gradient of the common cold is very limited.

Abnormal white blood cell counts, elevated C-reactive protein, bacteraemia or antibody levels indicate where to place the case on the *paraclinical gradient* of an inflammation process or immunological state.

Some disease manifestations may reflect both disease gradients and spectrums, such as an *in situ* growth, a metastatic spread and other components of cancer staging.

Contemporary medical literature abounds with the subject of *clinimetric indexes*. Some of these measure the spectrum and gradient of a single disease. Others do the same while covering a larger set of diseases and states, and yet others help to accurately categorize cases from among competing diagnoses. The *Glasgow Coma Scale*, the *Apgar Score*, the *Injury Severity Score (ISS)*, the *APACHE system (Acute Physiology and Chronic Health*

Evaluation) and the *Canadian Neurological Scale* are just a few examples.

These indexes should be carefully chosen and interpreted. Recommendations on how to do so have already been outlined in the clinical epidemiological literature[24,25,36] and are well beyond the scope of this reading.

Clinical and paraclinical data. Some states may be measured clinically or paraclinically. By way of example, physical examinations and haematological and biochemical findings may both be used to study malnutrition. Since space is generally limited in case reporting, clinical and paraclinical data should be chosen and reported as complementary parts of the case picture rather than as simple duplicate measurements of the same problem.

Co-morbidity. Depending on the problem under study, co-morbidity and its treatment may require a study and a presentation as precise as those of the disease of principal interest. This would help define the interactions between the former and the latter.

Diagnostic procedures, treatment intervention and care. In a clinical case report, the information being presented is almost always limited by time, if the communication is verbal, or by space, if the communication is presented in a journal. However, whenever the reader requires certain details in order to understand the risks, consequences, complications or successes in the management of the case, all clinical and paraclinical manoeuvres should be included in the clinical case study protocol and selectively presented in the report.

Expected as well as unexpected actions and events should be recorded. Intercurrent disorders and their treatment and the reasons for reporting them should also be outlined.

Outcome reporting focuses solely on the main outcome of interest. In other types of recording, *webs of consequences and outcomes* merit attention. For example, a psychiatrist might want to know not only about the drug abuser's sensorium, mood or cognitive functioning, but also about the patient's malnutrition, infections, marital and occupational problems, or delinquency. Is the reporting of these details necessary for a reasonable understanding of the case?

End-point of the case. Should the case report end at the moment of discharge from the hospital? Should events leading up to the admission and those occurring after the discharge be described in the case report? It is up to the case reporter to decide.

To summarize, an overall clinimetric description of the case should have qualities similar to those prized in writing and playing music[36]: movements creating a good component structure (disease stages), melody (construct validity, i.e. necessary components are like notes in a musical composition), harmony (clinical spectrum), dynamics (disease gradient) and rhythm (frequency, amplitude, and duration of disease spells and remissions).

In lieu of a conclusion, Table 5.6 outlines the clinical epidemiological challenges of case studies and reporting, including related precautions which should be known to the reporter and reader (and put into practice, if needed). *Obviously, all this information does not necessarily have to appear in the report. The author should nevertheless be ready to answer any questions raised regarding these matters.*

Discussion and conclusion

In this section, the author analyses the findings from his case, presents his conclusions and gives his *recommendations* for future work. These points are usually covered at the three levels illustrated in Table 5.7.

Three important questions must be answered in the discussion and conclusion section:
- What conclusions can be drawn from all the data obtained from the case?
- How can a synthesis of the case be produced in view of the actual experience illustrated by the case?
- What future actions should be taken in the light of this experience?

Let us now comment on the three points described in Table 5.7.

Discussion of observations and results – possible consequences of the case experience. As in any other scientific paper, this is the only section where the author has the freedom to express

Table 5.6 'The Twelve Commandments': Clinimetric criteria, rules and precautionary measures relevant to clinical case reporting

Clinimetric criteria and challenges	Precautionary measures
• Past and present risk characteristics of the patient	*Make clear distinctions between characteristics which can be modified (risk factors) and characteristics that can't (risk markers). Choose only those characteristics that are relevant to the case under study.*
• Clinical data and information	*Treat clinical data (measurements) and information (interpretations) as separate entities. Choose only data and information that are relevant to the diagnosis.*
• Criteria for clinical data and information	*Clearly define the diagnostic criteria and make them operational. Clearly distinguish between normalcy and abnormality. Usually, conceptual criteria are insufficient.*
• Syndrome and disease; two different clinical entities	*A syndrome is a syndrome and a disease is a disease. A syndrome is a set of often dissimilar manifestations common to several causes, diagnostic entities and aetiologies known or unknown, that do not necessarily lead to treatment. A disease is an entity (contrary to the above) with a distinct manifestation, cause, and treatment.*
• Clear notions of clinical signs, symptoms, and other phenomena	*In different circumstances and situations, the same clinical manifestation can be observed and recorded either as a sign (objective) or as a symptom (subjective).*

Table 5.6 continued

Clinimetric criteria and challenges	Precautionary measures
• Appropriate preservation of hard and soft data	*An attempt should be made to harden soft data whenever possible and the method of hardening should be known (definition, direction, analogy, recording.*
• Description of disease course (evolution of the case)	*Specify whether the description is based on the disease spectrum (extent), the disease gradient (severity), or both. Choose the best clinimetric indexes for measuring disease severity whenever a directional disease measurement is necessary.*
• Follow-up and recording of information regarding clinical and paraclinical procedures	*Always note the frequency, intensity, quality, quantity, and hierarchic organization of diagnostic (serial or parallel testing) and therapeutic manoeuvres.*
• Evaluation of the effect of a diagnostic or therapeutic manoeuvre	*Determine and be aware of the internal and external validity of the diagnostic procedures used, as well as their impact on clinical decision-making (treatment or no treatment, further diagnostic work-up, etc.). If known, keep in mind the effectiveness of preventive and therapeutic interventions in terms of aetiological and prognostic fractions.*
• Actions chosen which have clinical consequences and which influence diagnostic or therapeutic results	*The treatment and outcome of a disease require the same rigorous definition and description as does the presentation of this disease, its progress, and management. Try harden soft data whenever possible.*

Table 5.6 continued

● Prognostic characteristics	*Make clear distinctions between risk characteristics and prognostic characteristics. Specify the prognostic markers (non-modifiable) and the prognostic factors (modifiable).*
● Follow-up of co-morbid states and their treatment	*A rigorous and detailed study of co-morbidity and treatment of co-morbidity is necessary for a better understanding of differential diagnosis and preferred and adopted therapeutic decisions. The clinical and paraclinical management of all relevant morbid states should be equally well known, described, analysed, and explained.*

N.B. Other details and fundamental notions of clinimetrics can be found in textbooks devoted exclusively to clinical epidemiology and clinimetrics.

Table 5.7 – Components of the discussion and conclusion

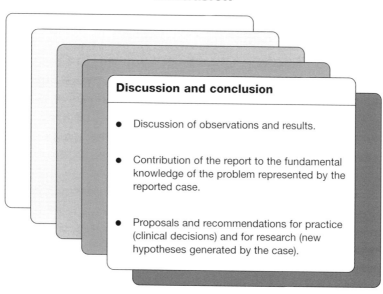

Discussion and conclusion

● Discussion of observations and results.

● Contribution of the report to the fundamental knowledge of the problem represented by the reported case.

● Proposals and recommendations for practice (clinical decisions) and for research (new hypotheses generated by the case).

criticisms, doubts and questions related to reported observations. Such a display of 'enlightened uncertainty' should help the reader understand the scope and range of the conclusions. Presenting confronting ideas in this section is also an option.

Any part of the case follow-up that might cause confusion or uncertainty, or require special attention, or represent an unusual observation should be highlighted.

There are two stages and levels of discussion based on the following questions:

- What is of interest solely in terms of this case report? This is a *within the case discussion*.
- What is of interest in a context larger than the case itself? This is a *beyond the case discussion*.

This section often takes up as much space as the case presentation itself, especially if the authors want (and they should):

- to compare their case with other cases of interest reported in the past;
- to specify the contribution of this case observation to the basic understanding of the disease or situation illustrated by the case.

Contribution of the case to the basic knowledge of the problem under study. What elements are helpful in understanding the problem and its fundamental mechanisms in terms of pathology, physiology, etc.? Can the pharmacodynamics of a given drug treatment be better understood? What are the morphologic or functional consequences of surgery? All these questions require answers.

What is 'new' and therefore worthy of discussion? Any phenomenon that has not yet been evaluated and elucidated in a given context as described in the case. For example, in the area of medical technology, any technology can be considered 'new' if its safety, efficacy and effectiveness, cost-effectiveness and cost–benefit ratios, and ethical, legal and social impact are unknown.

Proposals and recommendations for practice and research. To avoid unjustified generalizations, the analysis of a case must remain limited. The term **idiographic** analysis[37] was proposed for an analysis which is exclusive (or limited) to the case under study. This kind of analysis and its related recommendations also apply to the clinical case report.

However, special consideration should be given if the case is important for the basic sciences or for practical clinical purposes. Does the case represent a situation that requires more highly focused decisions? Is the case experience also important beyond the field of health sciences? Are there possible technological, social, cultural or economic implications?

Several obstacles stand in the way of tempting generalizations based on the single case, such as the obviously different demographic, biological and social characteristics of the patients, the severity of the cases, the co-morbidity and its treatment, the different treatments preferred by different physicians, the different care provided, the different migration of cases from one service or institution to another, and the admission policies.

For example, if a near fatal reaction is observed after a patient suffering from cardiac arrest is administered a sympathomimetic drug, its report alone does not warrant a contraindication right away. This observation should lead instead to a pharmacoepidemiological study (e.g. case–control study) which would demonstrate more clearly if such treatment in similar situations should be continued or rejected, given that the adverse effects have just been proved more effectively.

If differential diagnosis challenges are illustrated by the case, this should be a focus of the section. If difficult choices between competing treatments are reported, discussion and recommendations related to this problem should be included. Are rather unexpected complications and effects of treatment important? The reader does not necessarily know if they are, but should be told.

Do we always have to arrive at pragmatic conclusions? This depends. It is certainly important to present an unusual case and, if other similar cases appear, an epidemiological occurrence study of this phenomenon should be considered. Other cases are added to complete numerators, and community data provide denominators for rates of events of interest, which can be interpreted by epidemiological standards. Such uses may justify the multiplication of messages from various cases, ultimately leading to other pragmatic conclusions.

If prognostic or risk factors are of special interest in a case report, an adequate operational meaning should be given to them whenever necessary information is available. For example, a given treatment might be considered effective and a good prognostic factor. What do we know about the treatment's effectiveness beyond this case, or in other cases and situations? How might we reassess our treatment of the case in the light of such additional information?

Do we know something about the drug or surgery under study in terms of the following three points?

1. What is its **absolute risk reduction (ARR)**[44,45] power, i.e. the absolute arithmetic difference in the bad event rates (i.e. undesirable events such as non-responsiveness to treatment, complications, death etc.) of untreated and treated subjects ($Rate_{untreated} - Rate_{treated}$)? This measure is known to epidemiologists as the *attributable risk (AR)* or *risk difference (RD)*[36,46]. It shows what the true rate of bad events in untreated individuals is, since these subjects did not benefit from the treatment under study.

2. What is its **relative risk reduction (RRR)**[44,45] power, i.e. the proportional reduction in rates of bad events between control and experimental participants in a trial? This measure is known to epidemiologists as the *aetiologic fraction (EF)*, *attributable fraction (AF)*, *attributable risk per cent (AR%)*, or *protective efficacy rate (PER)*[36,46]. It shows what proportion of an overall rate of bad events in untreated subjects would be avoided if untreated subjects benefited from treatment: ($Rate_{untreated} - Rate_{treated} / Rate_{untreated}$) × 100. A result of 0 per cent shows no protective efficacy or relative risk reduction. A result of 100 per cent indicates absolute efficacy, i.e. treatment would prevent bad events in all untreated cases.

3. What does the **number needed to treat (NNT)**[44,45,47,48] mean for the use of this drug? This measure indicates the number of patients who need to be treated to achieve one additional favourable outcome. It is calculated as 1/ARR. If the clinician

knows an individual patient's specific baseline risk (patient expected event rate) or **F**, an NTT for the specific patient may be calculated as NNT/F[45].

When the treatment increases the probability of a good event, an **absolute benefit increase (ABI)** instead of the ARR and a **relative benefit increase (RBI)** instead of the RRR may be estimated. When the treatment increases the probability of a bad event, **absolute risk increase (ARI), relative risk increase (RRI)**, and the **number needed to harm (NNH)** may be also calculated[45].

When the role of a particular prognostic or risk factor in a clinical case report is discussed, this may be done by creating an analogy related to other situations and experiences reported in the literature in the above-mentioned terms.

If a treatment works in a single case, we can only guess that an outcome of interest is really due to this particular treatment. This should be confirmed by an analogous experience, extraneous to the case under study.

In summary, we might be interested if the diagnostic and therapeutic decisions surrounding the case are evidence-based. Also, this approach might indicate which interesting risk or prognostic factors in a single case should be evaluated by a more powerful method of gathering evidence in the future.

> Hence, choosing and presenting valid clinical and paraclinical data in a single case report is fundamental as a basis for evidence. Critically discussing the case from the point of view of the evidence in the literature and making conclusions based on the same principles progressively leads us to **evidence-based clinical case reporting**.

References

Like the other sections of the case report, the references should also be limited in terms of contents. The number of references should be reduced in such a way that only those references required for the basic understanding of the message should be cited. One reference covering the specific problem under study and another more general source are sometimes an acceptable minimum. One review article and some other references necessary to understand the contradictions between the findings from this case and those from other reports are also suitable.

Table 5.8 shows that references should cover three areas: the disease or problem under study, the clinical actions, and the decisions to be considered after this case experience.

One of the frequent problems with references is that they often cover just one of the three categories stated. For example, the reader may want to further study the disease, but he may not know where to start expanding his knowledge of clinical manoeuvres or complex decision points. Everything depends on the focus of the case report.

Recapitulation and synthesis

Once all the above-mentioned stages are complete, the organization and structure of a case report should follow the guidelines in Table 5.9.

Table 5.8 – The area references should cover

References

- Health problem and disease under study.

- Clinical and paraclinical actions.

- Decisions and actions under consideration.

Table 5.9 Architecture of the clinical case report

Summary*	• Motives and reasons for the report. *'Why are we reporting this?'* • Background to the problem. *'In what context?'* • Highlights of the report. *'What have we found?'* • Conclusions *'What does this mean?'*
Introduction	• Definition of the topic (problem, disease, clinical activity). • General context of the topic (relevant knowledge, present clinical situation and challenges). • A question that this report should answer or a gap in knowledge this report can fill. • Objectives and justification of this report.
Presentation of the case	• Situation, context and triggering factor of the report. • Clinical and paraclinical initial state of the patient. • Evolution of the clinical and paraclinical spectrum and gradient of the case. • Diagnostic and therapautic acts, care and support. • Expected and actual results of actions carried out or omitted. • Unexpected results and events.
Discussion and conclusion	• Discussion of observations and results. • Contribution of the report to the fundamental knowledge of the problem represented by the reported case. • Proposals and recommendations for practice (clinical decisions) and for research (new hypotheses generated by the case).
References	• Health problem and disease under study. • Clinical and paraclinical actions. • Decisions and actions under consideration.

*N.B. A summary of a clinical case report is not required by all medical journals.

The art of clinical case reporting relies on the author's wise selection of data and information, and on his/her ability to reduce and compress them within an allotted space. He/she must carefully balance the length of each section without losing the essential content of the message.

The underlying process is similar to the task assigned to Hermes in Greek mythology, whereby he had to interpret the gods' messages and make them understandable for humans. In other words, Hermes had to transform something from unintelligibility to understanding[49]. This is also the purpose of a case report: to draw out the most essential information from a maze of clinical data.

5.2.2.4 Form of a clinical case report

How can one respect all the rules of reporting and still fit all five sections of Table 5.9 into the required formats of the medical literature?

There are two prevailing attitudes in the area of clinical case reporting. On the one hand, periodicals prefer to publish only truly exceptional cases. If this is the situation, they are ready to offer as much space as needed. For example, the *Journal of the American Medical Association (JAMA)* has in the past devoted two full pages to a valuable clinical case report. On the other hand, case reports that are a more regular component of an issue are usually limited to between 500[50] and 1500 words (seven or eight double-spaced pages for some[51–53], four[54,55], six[18] or ten[56] pages for others). In addition, not more than three authors' names, three to six key words, two figures or tables, and five[51] to fifteen[53] references can be included.

According to the editors of *The Canadian Medical Association Journal*[55], '*a case report should comprise a title page, a 1000 word summary, an introduction, the case report, comments and references, and normally not exceed 800 words* (four double-spaced pages), *excluding the title page and references*'.

The case report must be written in simple, precise and concise language. Jargon, clichés, professional 'barbarisms', illogicalities and fashionable buzz-words, as well as 'lumpiness' of terms, should be avoided[10,51].

Let us also remember that presentations of rounds must adhere to the same rules[57].

Ethics and confidentiality must underlie any case report. A case titled 'Hip replacement at the Vatican for the leader of one of the world's major religions' demonstrates the author's lack of mastery of both above-mentioned virtues.

5.3 GENERAL AND SPECIFIC EXPECTATIONS OF MEDICAL JOURNALS FOR CASE REPORTS

Clinical case reports should conform to the same rules as other medical articles[58–60]. Checklists[61] can help achieve this goal.

As paradoxical as it may seem, a case report should address and explain similar issues to those encountered in review articles[62]. These issues generally relate to the reasons for the report, the sources of information, the rules governing the selection and presentation of information, the valid materials, the systematic gathering of data, the review of possible limitations and inconsistencies, the summary, and the recommendations.

Table 5.10 summarizes the *Canadian Medical Association Journal* expectations with regard to case reports[17]. The reader should also refer to Tables 5.1 and 5.9 as additional guides in preparing his/her own clinical case presentation.

5.4 IN CONCLUSION

A clinical case report is an endeavour as serious as any other article or scientific paper in medicine. Its content and form should live up to the expectations that are now clearly stated in many medical journals. Let us respect these expectations.

A last word of advice to future medical casuists. The required brevity of clinical case reports is not an excuse for hiding erroneous or missing data and findings. Good data and information, often beyond the scope of the case report, should always be at hand. In fact, they are essential[47,63,64]. The ability to produce a

Table 5.10 CMAJ expectations with regards to case reports (reproduced with kind permission of *The Canadian Medical Association Journal*)

Summary

- Does the summary give a succinct description of the case and its implications?

Introduction

- Is the case new or uncommon, with important public health implications?
- Is the rationale for reporting the case adequately explained?
- Has an adequate review of the literature been done?

Description of the case

- Is the case described briefly but comprehensively?
- Is the case described clearly?
- Are the results of investigations and treatments described adequately, including doses, schedule and duration of treatment?
- Are the results of less common laboratory investigations accompanied by normal values?

Comments

- Is the evidence to support the author's diagnosis presented?
- Are other plausible explanations considered and refuted?
- Are the implications and relevance of the case discussed?
- Is the evidence to support the author's recommendations presented adequately?
- Does the author indicate directions for further investigation or management of similar cases?

concise, to the point presentation is mainly an acquired, learned and mastered skill.

Independent of the case report's length, it should result from a serious in-depth qualitative analysis.

Psychiatric and psychoanalytic work-ups and evaluations[65], patient follow-ups and case presentations are hermeneutic and phenomenologic processes[66] *par excellence*.

A clinical casuist observes, measures, records and establishes a **theory**; i.e. he/she selects an *interrelated set of constructs (or variables) formed into propositions or hypotheses that specify the relationship*

CLINICAL CASE REPORTING

between variables[66]. These variables must be carefully chosen. Not all of them are necessary, depending on the purpose of the study. If aetiology is the focus of attention, variables constituting a possible network of causes must be evaluated. If prognosis is the main subject, variables constituting possible networks of consequences should be taken into consideration. If possible sources of confusion such as co-morbidity, treatment for co-morbidity etc. are important, they should be included in the observation or interpretation of the case.

Consequently, as already mentioned in Section 5.2.2.3 under 'presentation of the case', a case report is methodologically based on a blend of qualitative research from its conception[67] to its presentation[68], and on clinimetrics[24–26]. It also supports recent endeavours to integrate qualitative and quantitative research methods[69].

Certainly, clinical case reporting is the weakest step in the lines of medical evidence of causes. However, it is also medicine's first rate evidence **of what happened**, so it is that much more important for the case report to be right. If the report is based on a disorganized and unfocused approach, and poor and incomplete observations, recordings, analyses and interpretations, it is of little value. The challenge is to create a report in such a way that building stronger evidence based on the case report is worth the effort.

A clinical case report cannot extend beyond its own purposes, namely to explore, describe, explain and raise questions. This fact is even more important given that many new challenges have originated from case reports: genetic disorders and mapping, organ transplantation, microsurgery, *in vitro* fertilization, cloning, genetically engineered vaccines and drugs etc. Stronger evidence of the *raison d'être* of such new technologies has usually followed.

Even a case report, despite its own inherent limitations, must:

- have an acceptable focus (problem and question);
- be sound;
- be well-structured;
- be based on a known process; and
- be specific and clear for the reader, in terms of its message.

Moreover, any researcher can surpass the efforts of a clinical case reporter by building on his or her own case experience by planning and undertaking a study of numerous cases in a case series report or in an occurrence study (a descriptive study in epidemiological terms) or by comparing two or more groups in explanatory research.

If the next lines of evidence in medicine rely on a poorly selected index case, the whole process of producing evidence is at high risk of being diverted along the wrong path.

It is hoped that this chapter illustrates at least in part that the whole exercise of clinical case reporting extends far beyond an intern's wish to 'just survive' his/her case presentation[70].

Does the reader now need to temporarily escape from this Cartesian approach to clinical case reporting? A funnier, but eloquent, review of case report thinking in Bennett's book[71] is an uplifting remedy for the reader's probable state of mind. When the reader does pick up this text again, Chapter 6 will present an example of a good clinical case report. Chapter 7 will then show how to report a set of cases as a clinical case series report.

REFERENCES

1. Yurchak PM. A guide to medical case presentations. *Res Staff Phys*, 1981 (September); **27**: 109–15.
2. Zack BG. A guide to pediatric case presentations. *Res Staff Phys*, 1982 (November); **28**: 71–80.
3. Pickell GC. The oral case presentation. *Res Staff Phys*, 1987(June); **33**: 141–5.

4. Locante J. The anatomy of a perfect case presentation: A–Z. *J Oral Implantol*, 1996; **XXII**: 65–7.

5. Huth EJ. The case report (Chapter 6, pp. 58–63) and The review and the case-series analysis (Chapter 7, pp. 64–68) in: *How to Write and Publish Papers in the Medical Sciences*. Philadelphia: iSi Press, 1982. (See also 2nd Edition. Baltimore: Williams & Wilkins, 1990.)

6. Simpson RJ Jr, Griggs TR. Case reports and medical progress. *Persp Biol Med*, 1985 (Spring); **28**: 402–6.

7. Coates M-M. Writing for publication: Case reports. *J Hum Lact*, 1992; **8**: 23–6.

8. Freeman TR. The patient-centred case presentation. *Fam Pract*, 1994; **11**: 164–70.

9. DeBakey L, DeBakey S. The case report. I. Guidelines for preparation. *Int J Cardiol*, 1983; **4**:3 57–64.

10. DeBakey L, DeBakey S. The case report. II. Style and form. *Int J Cardiol*, 1984; **6**: 247–54.

11. Kroenke K. The case presentation. Stumbling blocks and stepping stones. *Am J Med*, 1985; **79**: 605–8.

12. Mott T Jr. Guidelines for writing case reports for the hypnosis literature. *Am J Clin Hypnosis*, 1996; **29**: 1–6.

13. Lilleyman JS. How to write a scientific paper – rough guide to getting published. *Arch Dis Childhood*, 1995; **72**: 268–270.

14. Levin M. How to write a case report. *Res Staff Phys*, 1998; **44**(1): 60–3.

15. Squires BP. Case reports: What editors want from authors and peer reviewers. *Can Med Assoc J*, 1989; **141**: 379–80.

16 Squires BP, Elmslie TJ. Reports of case series: What editors expect from authors and peer reviewers. *Can Med Assoc J*, 1990; **142**: 1205–6.

17. Huston P. Squires BP. Case reports: Information for authors and peer reviewers. *Can Med Assoc J*, 1996; **154**: 43–4.

18. Riesenberg DE. Case reports in the medical literature. *JAMA*, 1986; **255**: 2067.

19. *Landmark Articles in Medicine*. Edited by HS Meyer and GD Lundberg. Chicago: American Medical Association, 1985.

20. Levine P, Stetson RE. An unusual case of intra-group agglutination. *JAMA*, 1939; **113**:126–7. (Reprinted in: *JAMA*, 1984; **251**: 1316–7.)

21. Levine P, Newark NJ, Burnham L, Englewood NJ, Katzin EM, Vogel P. The role of isoimmunization in the pathogenesis of erythroblastosis fetalis. *Am J Obstet Gynecol*, 1941; **42**: 925–37.

22. Greenwalt TJ. Rh isoimmunization. The importance of a critical case study. *JAMA*, 1984; **251**: 1318–20.

23. DeBakey L, DeBakey S. The case report. I. Guidelines for preparation. *Int J Cardiol*, 1983; **4**: 357–64.

24. Feinstein AR. *Clinical Epidemiology. The Architecture of Clinical Research*. Philadelphia: WB Saunders, 1985 (p. 241).

25. Feinstein AR. *Clinimetrics*. New Haven and London: Yale University Press, 1987.

26. Jenicek M. *Epidemiology. The Logic of Modern Medicine*. Montreal: Epimed International, 1995.

27. Kahn CR. Picking a research problem. The critical decision. *N Engl J Med*, 1994; **330**: 1530–3.

28. *How to Conduct a Cochrane Systematic Review*, 3rd Edition. Edited by CM Mulrow and A Oxman. San Antonio: San Antonio Cochrane Center, 1996.

29. Counsell C. Formulating questions and locating primary studies for inclusion in systematic reviews. *Ann Intern Med* 1997; 127: 380–7.

30. Yackee J, Lipson A, Wasserman AG. Electrocardiographic changes suggestive of cardiac ischemia in a patient with esophageal food impaction. 'A case that's hard to swallow'. *JAMA*, 1986; **255**: 2065–6.

31. Haynes RB, Mulrow CD, Huth EJ, Altman DG, Gardner MJ. More informative abstracts revisited. *Ann Intern Med*, 1990; **113**: 69–76

32. Mulrow CD, Thacker SB, Pugh JA. A proposal for more informative abstracts of review articles. *Ann Intern Med*, 1988; **108**: 613–5

33. *Ad Hoc* Working Group for Critical Appraisal of the Medical Literature (Haynes RB *et al.*). A proposal for more informative abstracts of clinical articles. *Ann Intern Med*, 1987; **106**: 598–604

34. Richtsmeier WJ. Case report. *Arch Otolaryngol Head Neck Surg*, 1993; **119**: 926.

35. Nahum AM. The case report: 'Pot boiler' or scientific literature? *Head Neck Surg*, 1979; **1**: 291–2.

36. Jenicek M. Making clinical pictures or describing disease in an individual, Section 5.2, pp. 125–136 in: *Epidemiology. The Logic of Modern Medicine.* Montreal: Epimed International, 1995.

37. Barr JE. Research and writing basics: Elements of the case study. *Ostomy/Wound Management*, 1995; **41**(1): 18, 20, 21.

38. Weiss K, Laverdière M. *Salmonella typhi* osteomyelitis in an immunocompetent patient. *Clin Microbiol Newsletter*, 1995; **17**: 35–6.

39. Kamarulzaman A, Briggs RJS, Fabinyi G, Richards MJ. Skull osteomyelitis due to *Salmonella* species: Two case reports and review. *Clin Infect Dis*, 1996; **22**: 638–41.

40. *A Dictionary of Epidemiology*, 3rd Edition. Edited by JM Last. Oxford and New York: Oxford University Press, 1995.

41. Feinstein AR. *Clinimetrics*. New Haven: Yale University Press, 1987.

42. Rothe JP. *Qualitative Research. A Practical Guide.* Heidelberg and Toronto: RCI/PDE Publications, 1993.

43. Feinstein AR. *Clinical Biostatistics*. St Louis: CV Mosby, 1977.

44. Sackett DL, Richardson WS, Rosenberg W, Haynes RB. Evidence-based medicine. How to practice and teach EBM. New York: Churchill Livingstone, 1997.

45. Anon. Evidence-based medicine. Glossary. *Evidence-Based Med*, 1999 (May/June); **4**: inside back cover.

46. Jenicek M. Epidemiology, evidence-based medicine, and evidence-based public health. *J Epidemiol*, 1997; **7**: 187–97.

47. Laupacis A, Sackett DL, Roberts RS. An assessment of clinically useful measures of the consequences of treatment. *N Engl J Med*, 1988; **318**: 1728–33.

48. Chatellier G, Zapletal E, Lemâitre D, Ménard J, Degoulet P. The number

needed to treat: a clinically useful nomogram in its proper context. *BMJ*, 1996; **312**: 426–9.

49. Addison RB. Grounded hermeneutic research, pp. 110–124 in: *Doing Qualitative Research*. Edited by BJ Crabtree and WL Miller. Newbury Park: Sage Publications, 1992.

50. Information for authors. *Intern J Cardiol*, 1995; **51**: 309–10.

51. Soffer A. Case reports in the Archives of Internal Medicine. *Arch Intern Med*, 1976; **136**: 1090.

52. Mott T Jr. Guidelines for writing case reports for the hypnosis literature. *Am J Clin Hypnosis*, 1986; **29**: 1–6.

53. Information for contributors. *Urology*, 1994; **44**: 153–N.

54. Information for authors. *Surgery*, 1994; **115**: 7A–8A.

55. Instructions for authors. *Can Med Assoc J*, 1995, **152**: 55–7.

56. Instructions for contributors. *Am J Respir Crit Care Med*, 1995, **152**:1/95–3/95.

57. Winter R. Edit a staff round. *Br Med J*, 1991; **303**: 1258–9.

58. Lilleyman JS. How to write a scientific paper – a rough guide to getting published. *Arch Dis Childhood*, 1995; **72**: 268–70.

59. Skelton J. Analysis and structure of original research papers: an aid to writing original papers for publication. *Br J Gen Practice*, 1994; **44**: 455–9.

60. International Committee of Medical Journal Editors. Uniform requirements for manuscripts submitted to biomedical journals. *Ann Intern Med*, 1997; **126**: 36–47.

61. DuRant RH. Checklist for the evaluation of research articles. *J Adolesc Health*, 1994; **15**: 4–8.

62. Milne R, Chambers L. Assessing the scientific quality of review articles. *J Epidemiol Comm Med*, 1993; **47**: 169–70.

63. Weed LL. Medical records that guide and teach. *N Engl J Med*, 1968; **278**:593–600. (Concluded in: *N Engl J Med*, 1968; **278**: 652–7.)

64. Koran LM. The reliability of clinical methods, data and judgements. *N Engl J Med*, 1975; **293**:642–6. (Continued in: *N Engl J Med*, 1975; **293**: 695–701.)

65. Shea SC. *Psychiatric Interviewing. The Art of Understanding*, 2nd Edition. Philadelphia: WB Saunders, 1998.

66. Creswell JW. *Research Design. Qualitative and Quantitative Approaches*. Thousand Oaks: Sage Publications, 1994.

67. Kuckelman Cobb A, Nelson Hagemaster J. Ten criteria for evaluating qualitative research proposals. *J Nurs Educ*, 1987; **26**: 138–43.

68. Forchuk C, Roberts J. How to critique qualitative research articles. *Can J Nurs Res*, 1993; **25**(4): 47–55.

69. Stange KC, Miller WL, Crabtree BF, O'Connor PJ, Zyzanski SJ. Multimethod research: approaches for integrating qualitative and quantitative methods. *J Gen Intern Med*, 1994; **9**: 278–82.

70. Bennett HJ. How to survive a case presentation. *Chest*, 1985; **88**: 292–4.

71. Case reports, pp. 117–135 in: *The Best of Medical Humor. A Collection of Articles, Essays, Poetry, and Letters Published in the Medical Literature*, 2nd Edition. Compiled and Edited by HJ Bennett. Philadelphia: Hanley & Belfus, Inc., 1997.

CHAPTER 6

Annotated
example of a
clinical case
report

CHAPTER 6

Is there really an example of a good clinical single case report that meets the stringent criteria mentioned above? Certainly, we have found at least one!

Annotated example of a clinical case report

6.1 INTRODUCTION TO THE EXAMPLE

The principles and requirements of a good clinical case report as reviewed in Chapter 5 should be followed in all clinical case reports in the literature. In reality, many reports are excellent and many are not. From the former pool, we have chosen one[1].

Yackee, Lipson and Wasserman have reported electrocardiographic changes as a challenge of differential diagnosis between an oesophageal impaction and coronary ischaemia[1]. Their case report elicited two important editorial comments. Riesenberg[2] discusses a framework of good editorial policies regarding clinical case reports. Swirin and Hueter[3] analyse differential diagnostic challenges in situations where both cardiovascular and digestive disorders must be considered. To save space, these comments are not reproduced here. The reader is encouraged to find them in the literature[2,3] as suggested additional reading.

The pages that follow are an intact reproduction (with permission) of Yackee et al.'s report. In our own step by step annotations, places where good elements of a clinical case report have been put into practice have been underlined. We have also mentioned some missing points and possible areas of improvement. This, however, should not devalue in any way the authors' endeavour.

This clinical case report is worthy of attention for several reasons. First, the authors present an unexpected event. Then, they compare it to cases where electrocardiographic abnormalities were observed in conjunction with other digestive disorders. Finally, the authors discuss the practical implications for clinical decisions in similar situations. Obviously, this report has a well-structured, logical sequence that is easy to follow and grasp.

Relevant elements of the report are indicated by a graphic symbol (open square) corresponding to an identical sideline pictogram and related comments.

There should be enough page space to allow the reader to add his or her own comments and points to ponder. This interactive reading is strongly encouraged. Our comments are neither complete nor a reflection of the absolute truth. Work with this example while reading it!

Reminder: The case report reproduced here is a methodological example only. It is not in any way indicative of clinical diagnostic, therapeutic or prognostic decisions, which may change in time with increasing knowledge in the field under consideration.

6.2 ANNOTATED CASE REPORT

Electrocardiographic Changes Suggestive of Cardiac Ischemia in a Patient With Esophageal Food Impaction.

'A Case That's Hard to Swallow'*

John Yackee, MD, Ace Lipson, MD, Allan G. Wasserman, MD*

□Many patients presenting with chest pain initially believed to be cardiac in etiology may, in fact, have esophageal disease as an alternative or additional cause of their complaints. □Although electrocardiographic (ECG) repolarization abnormalities have been well described in gastroenterologic processes, such as pancreatitis and cholecystitis[1], and have been reported in esophageal disease[2-9], the ECG is generally thought to be a reliable means of distinguishing between esophageal and cardiac pain[10,11]. □In this report we describe a patient who developed ECG changes suggestive of cardiac ischemia secondary to esophageal food impaction.

□The clinical revelance of the topic is high-lighted.

□References to the literature summarize the overall knowledge of the problem as well as prevailing practices and decisions in similar circumstances.

□Objectives of this case report are stated here. (why the case is reported)

Report of a case

□A 57-year-old woman was admitted to the George Washington University Medical Center, Washington, DC, with a chief complaint of chest discomfort and dysphagia. She had a history of intermittent epigastric and substernal burning discomfort with meals, alleviated by antacids, and in 1979 was found to have a hiatal hernia with reflux by an upper gastrointestinal (GI) tract X-ray series. For

□The patient's medical history is outlined as it relates mainly to cardiology and gastroenterology, the areas of focus of the differential diagnosis of this case. The patient's 'initial state' (at admission) is also reported.

*Reprinted from *JAMA (Journal of the American Medical Association)*, 18 April 1986;255:2065–6. (Copyright 1986, American Medical Association. Reproduced with permission.)
** From the Division of Cardiology, Department of Medicine, George Washington University Medical Center, Washington, DC.

three to four years, she has noted intermittent dysphagia, with a sensation of solid foods 'sticking' in her throat. A repeated upper GI tract X-ray series 11 months before admission revealed the hiatal hernia with an area of mucosal irregularity in the distal esophagus, consistent with reflux esophagitis. She was managed with elevation of the head of her bed, antacids, thorough chewing of foods, and avoidance of caffeine and alcohol, with improvement. There was no history of exertional chest pain. On the day of admission, while eating steak at a dinner party after drinking several cocktails, she had the sensation of a piece of meat sticking in her throat, associated with subxyphoid and epigastric discomfort with a mild nausea and hiccoughs. She was unable to swallow liquids, regurgitating even her own oral secretions.

□Co-morbidity and treatment for co-morbidity are mentioned.

□Medical history included hypertension, manic-affective disorder, degenerative joint disease, aspiration pneumonia following a drug overdose, and excision of benign thyroid and breast nodules. Her medications included atenolol, 75mg/day, and antacids.

□Results of a clinical and paraclinical work-up at admission are presented as the patient's 'initial state' (e.g. ECG, radiography – see Figures 1 and 2).

□Physical examination revealed a calm, moderately obese woman regurgitating her saliva into a cup. Blood pressure was 120/70mmHg; heart rate 84 beats per minute and regular, respirations 18/min and unlabored. The cardiac and abdominal findings were unremarkable. Laboratory values were remarkable for a potassium level of 3.2mEq/l. Chest X-ray film was normal. The ECG taken on admission revealed ST-segment depression and T-wave inversion in the inferior and anterolateral leads (Figure 1), which had not been evident on previous

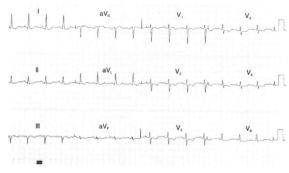

Figure 1 – Twelve-lead electrocardiogram during esophageal meat impaction. Note interior and anferolateral ST-segment depression and T-wave inversion

tracings. A barium swallow examination showed an irregularly contoured, intraluminal, esophageal filling defect proximal to the gastroesophageal junction (Figure 2).

☐Sublingual nitroglycerin and intravenous glucagon were administered, without resolution of symptoms.

Esophagoscopy revealed a large piece of meat impacted in the distal esophagus at 35cm. After administration of sublingual nifedipine, the meat bolus was mechanically advanced into the stomach.

☐Mucosal edema and superficial ulceration at the site of impaction, and a hiatal hernia distal to the site of impaction, were noted. There was no evidence of an esophageal stricture. An ECG obtained soon after endoscopic disimpaction showed marked improvement of the ST-T-wave changes (Figure 3).

☐Treatment according to the working diagnosis is defined and delivered (in order to exclude coronary co-morbidity), followed by the treatment (therapeutic manoeuvre) of the main problem under consideration (disimpaction of the oesophagus).

☐The 'subsequent state' of the patient is reported and confirmed by the paraclinical follow-up (ECG after disimpaction).

Comment

☐ST-wave abnormalities have been reported in association with hiatal hernia,[12] esophageal spasm,[2-5,7-9] epiphrenic esophageal diverticulum,[6] and experimental mechanical

☐Challenges of the differential diagnosis from the cardiology and gastroenterology points of view are given here with special attention to the ECG findings.

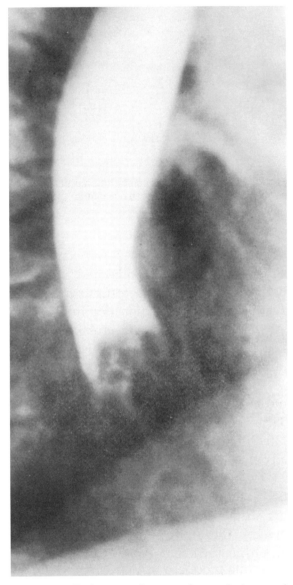

Figure 2 – Barium esophagram demonstrates meat bolus impacted in distal esophagus

distention of the esophagus.[10] However, we are aware of no other reported cases of ST-T-wave changes attributable to esophageal food impaction. This patient presented with chest discomfort and ECG changes consis-

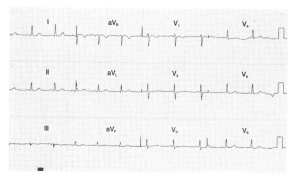

Figure 3 – Repeated 12-lead electrocardiogram after esophageal disimpaction. Note resolution of previous ST-T-wave changes

tent with cardiac ischemia. Although the history of previous esophageal symptoms, the subjective sensation of food lodging in the throat, and the upper GI tract X-ray and endoscopic findings make the esophageal etiology of her chest discomfort readily apparent, this case has important implications regarding the reliability of ECG changes in differentiating cardiac and esophageal causes of chest pain. This differentiation can otherwise be difficult since historical features and the character of chest pain in each can frequently be indistinguishable.[2] Both can be alleviated by similar therapy, such as nitrates or calcium blockers, or precipitated by provocation testing, such as with ergonovine or methacholine chloride,[5,8] and both processes can occur in the same patient.[4,7]

□Explanations for this patient's ECG findings other than esophageal disease seem unlikely. Since our patient did not undergo cardiac catheterization with ergonovine provocation, a cardiac etiology for the ECG changes, such as ischemia precipitated by the esophageal impaction, cannot be completely

□The authors justify and specify their final diagnosis.

excluded. However, the lack of previous cardiac history and the prompt resolution of the changes with esophageal disimpaction argue strongly against such a role of cardiac ischemia. The patient also has recently had normal results on a treadmill exercise test.

☐A differential diagnosis is discussed by exclusion on the basis of the patient's history. It is important to note that the patient's past manic-depressive disorder has not been omitted either.

☐Similarly, cardiac ischemia precipitated by coronary spasm as one component of a generalized disorder of smooth muscle, including a simultaneous esophageal motility disorder, seems unlikely.[7,8] The patient's history and ECG changes do not suggest coronary spasm.

Repolarization abnormalities have been reported in hiatal hernia[11] postprandially, with hypokalemia, anxiety, and psychiatric disorders, each of which might be invoked as playing a role in the present case. However, none of these is consistent with the patient's presentation, in particular, the transient appearance of the changes coincident with the development and resolution of the food impaction.

☐Underlying possible pathological/physiological mechanisms are discussed, which is proof that they have not been forgotten.

☐The mechanism by which esophageal meat impaction might cause ST-T-wave changes is speculative. A vagal mechanism for similar changes observed in gastroenterologic conditions, such as pancreatitis and cholecystitis, has been proposed. Since gag is a powerful vagal stimulus, it would not be surprising that esophageal obstruction might provide such a stimulus. A mechanical shift of the T-wave axis secondary to a direct effect seems unlikely given only a minor change in the QRS axis. It is also difficult to conceive how a direct mechanical effect due to the proximity of the esophagus to the heart might induce ventricular repolarization abnormalities.

□In conclusion, a patient with underlying esophageal disease and no evidence of coronary artery disease developed marked ST-T-wave changes with esophageal food impaction, resolving promptly with disimpaction.

□We believe this is the first reported case of ST-T-wave changes due to clinical esophageal impaction and speculate an autonomic esophageal–cardiac interplay as the mechanism. □This case provides additional evidence that the ECG is not always a reliable means of differentiating chest pain of cardiac and esophageal etiologies.

□A summary of the pathological/physiological findings is presented.

□The originality of the observations and findings as a justification for this case report is stressed.

□Decisions are proposed for similar situations in clinical practice.

□References

1. Schamroth L (ed); *The Electrocardiology of Coronary Artery Disease*, ed 2. London, Blackwell Scientific Publications Ltd, 1984.
2. Davies HA, Rhodes J: How often does the gut cause angina pain? *Acta Med Scand* 1981; 209(suppl 644): 62–65.
3. Dart AM, Davies AH, Loundes RH *et al.*: Oesophageal spasm and angina: Diagnostic value of ergometrine (ergonovine) provocation. *Eur Heart J* 1980; 1: 91–95.
4. Edeiken J: Angina pectoris and spasm of the cardia with pain of anginal distribution on swallowing. *JAMA* 1939; 112: 2272–2274.
5. Davis AH, Kaye MD, Rhodes J *et al.*: Diagnosis of oesophageal spasm by ergometrine provocation. *Gut* 1982; 23: 89–97.
6. Julian DG: Epiphrenic oesophageal diverticulum with cardiac pain. *Lancet* 1953; 2: 915–916.
7. Lee MG, Sullivan SN, Watson WC, *et al*: Chest pain: Esophageal, cardiac or both? *J Am Coll Cardiol* 1985; 80: 320–324.
8. Eastwood GL, Weiner BH, Dickerson WJ *et al.*: Use of ergonovine to identify esophageal spasm in patients with chest pain. *Ann Intern Med* 1981; 94: 768–771.
9. Davies HA, Jones DB, Rhodes J: Esophageal angina as a cause of chest pain. *JAMA* 1982; 248: 2274–2278.

□The references focus mainly on the challenge of differential diagnosis in similar situations of cardiac or digestive chest pain.

10. Baylis JH, Kauntze R, Trounce JR: Observations on distension of the lower esophagus. *Q J Med* 1955; 94: 143–153.
11. Kramer P, Hollander W: Comparison of experimental esophageal pain with clinical pain of angina pectoris and esophageal disease, *Gastroenterology* 1955; 29: 719–743.
12. Delmonico JE Jr, Black A, Geusini GG: Diaphragmatic hiatal hernia and angina pectoris. *Dis Chest* 1968; 53: 309–315.

6.3   CONCLUDING COMMENTS

This 'straight to the point' report from the Washington University authors led to other considerations in the two above-mentioned editorial comments[2,3].

Usually, clinical reports from North America focus on decisions and actions. In contrast, case reports from Europe generally stress the understanding of the underlying physiological and pathological mechanisms of the case and clinical problem under study.

In fact, it is the author's duty to highlight the uniqueness of the case and its relevance from the point of view of the basic sciences (e.g. anatomy, physiology, pathology, pharmacodynamics), as well as its usefulness for diagnostic and therapeutic clinical decisions and for prognosis.

Meeting all these requirements remains a great challenge, especially if the message has to be conveyed briefly to a somnolent colleague after a weekend, to a confused and disoriented freshman, or to an overburdened senior staff person.

Clinical case reports must become more focused and structured in order to facilitate the reader's understanding. Since the author is responsible for the quality of his or her report, he or she may want to refer back to Chapter 5 of this book, which should serve as a useful tune-up checklist for the emission (author) and the reception (readers).

Last but not least, to fulfil the clinical case report's purpose and objectives, more than the one or two customary paragraphs may be needed. If so, a stringent selection of case reports is needed to justify the precious space devoted to them in any current issue of a reputed medical journal.

The author and reader must always ask themselves if this report makes a contribution to the first line of evidence in medicine. If not, let us forget it.

A case report certainly represents a very limited contribution to evidence in medicine, but it is also precisely the point at which the cascade of evidence begins. Therefore, we must ensure that our case reports are prepared correctly.

REFERENCES

1. Yackee J, Lipson A, Wasserman AG. Electrocardiographic changes suggestive of cardiac ischemia in a patient with esophageal food impaction. 'A case that's hard to swallow'. *JAMA*, 1986; **255**: 2065–6.
2. Riesenberg DE. Case reports in the medical literature. *JAMA*, 1986; **255**: 2067.
3. Swiryn S, Hueter DC. The electrocardiogram in esophageal impaction. *JAMA*, 1986; **255**: 2067–8.

Assessing the evidence from multiple observations: case series reports and systematic reviews of cases

CHAPTER 7

Assessing the evidence from multiple observations: case series reports and systematic reviews of cases

Clinical case series are like the military cohorts at the time of the Roman Empire, marching steadily to an uncertain fate. However, it should be easier for us to predict our patient's outcome than the destiny of the warriors under the Centurions' commands.

7.1 WHAT ARE CLINICAL CASE SERIES?

As unusual and rare as some cases may be, they may actually reappear. For some, a case report is limited to one case only[1]. For others, two cases constitute a case report and three[2] to ten[3] cases or more make up a **case series**. Nevertheless, no rule governs the minimum number of cases that form a **set of cases** or a **case series**.

The study of more than one case has two main objectives:

- to determine the prevailing characteristics of a given set of patients; and/or
- to determine the prevailing outcomes for these patients.

For our assessment, let us state that *case series are very different from classical occurrence (descriptive) studies in epidemiology.* In occurrence studies, the number of cases is usually linked to some larger groups of individuals from which they originate. For example, if 10 cases of cancer in a given year are observed in a community of 100,000 subjects, this event may be presented as a **rate** of 10/100,000, where the numerator (10) relates to the denominator of 100,000. In our terms, *case series studies are studies of numerators only.* Denominators in case series studies are most often unknown or extremely difficult to define.

In addition to the 'numerator focus' of case series, only one set of patients is under study. No control group or controlled assignments of patients to clinical manoeuvres is involved. Case series, then, bear little resemblance to observational aetiological research or clinical trials.

It is also hard to ascertain if the assembled cases truly exist or if they are more or less representative of some other cases beyond our grasp.

Nevertheless, aside from these inherent limitations, case studies are often the only source of information about the problem of interest. Therefore, they must be correctly structured, observed, analysed and interpreted within their own limits. Case series are neither proofs of a cause (aetiology) nor proofs of efficacy or effectiveness of treatment (especially in cases when even historical controls are not available).

The presentation of a limited number of cases [4,5] indicates that the first case is probably not unique, and that a better descriptive study might or should be attempted. Such cases can be considered in epidemiological terms as **index cases**, beyond which the study should be expanded. Their presentation must be acceptable from the point of view of **clinimetrics**[6].

For example, Selzer[7] reports several cases of multiple personality. In psychiatry, as in toxicology, clinical microbiology or environmental studies, reports of a limited number of cases are often the only ones available.

Case series are usually presented in one of two forms:

- as review articles[8]; or
- as descriptive studies[9] with all the above-mentioned limitations.

Similarly to any other area of clinical and epidemiological research, case series studies must be prepared according to certain rules. The limitations of case series reports should not be used as an excuse to avoid the rigour of thought required for their presentation. In reality, problems generally arise as a result of the mediocrity of the author's work or the lack of skill displayed by the reader with regards to the reading and understanding of case series reports[10].

7.2 CLASSIFICATION OF CASE SERIES STUDIES

A

Case series studies may be classified in several ways, as outlined below.

1. **According to the origin of the cases.** The authors may:

- report cases that they have observed themselves; or
- assemble case series from several clinical sites; or
- assemble case series from the literature and present them either in a somewhat haphazard way or systematically as a kind of *'meta-analysis of cases'*.

2. **According to the number of case examinations in time.** The case series can represent:

- a *cross-sectional study*; i.e. an instant portrait of case characteristics; or
- a *longitudinal study*, usually based on a single cohort only. Repeated measurements in this situation allow a better understanding of the clinical course of cases and their outcomes.

3. **According to the number of case series involved.** In this situation:

- either one set of patients is studied in order to obtain their clinical portrait; or
- two or more case series may be compared in a framework of analytical, observational or quasi-experimental design (different treatments for each series etc.).

A combination of these three axes of classification may be found in each case series report and in the systematic review of cases/case series.

7.3 METHODOLOGICAL ASPECTS OF CASE SERIES REPORTS

For Huth[8], case series analyses are a kind of hybrid paper *'based on a retrospective study of case records, usually cases collected in one institution. The cases may be described in short case reports that are followed* by such generalizations as can be drawn from these cases and, perhaps, from similar cases in the literature. In this format the paper has much of the character of a single case report'. Other papers are written deductively; i.e. to answer some pre-study formulated question, in a form that is closer to more classical observational or experimental aetiological studies.

In general, a case series report is either a sort of a review article that conforms to the corresponding general rules[11] or an occurrence study as mentioned above.

7.3.1 Presenting case series and reviewing the literature

The order of presentation can vary. Either the problem is explained first (for example, pregnancy in Parkinson's disease[12]) and the case report (author's own experience) follows, or the reverse occurs. Although the latter situation is much more prevalent, both sequences are acceptable.

In general, the **presentation of cases** must follow the rules specified in Chapter 5 of this book.

The **review of the literature** is an additional methodological challenge. It should be based preferably on the **systematic review principles and methodology** outlined in other sources[13–15]. The review of the literature must be **evidence-based**, i.e. founded on a uniform and structured evaluation of original evidence from various sources (e.g. a MEDLINE search with terms used in the search), followed by an equally structured synthesis of findings and an assessment of the heterogeneous results obtained from original studies as a basis for clinical decision recommendations.

The review of the literature can cover the pathology under study and its management, or the methodology of the study, depending on the objectives, questions and focus of the case report or case series report. Journal editors should not be too miserly with their space if the literature review is well done.

7.3.2 Establishing a portrait of cases: cross-sectional descriptions

7.3.2.1 Reviewing and summarizing several cases

When regrouping several cases, as in any other systematic review, identical information should be sought and reported from one case to another. The basic information should be presented in the form of an **evidence table**, a technique well known to meta-analysts and to those involved in the systematic review of evidence in health care.

In such tables, the presence or absence of a preselected set of information is *systematically* compared from one clinical case to another whether the cases are from the same source, from multiple sources in the literature, or obtained through clinical case linkages with different hospitals, services etc.

This kind of **checklist of case characteristics** can be included in a cross-sectional study, as in Cole's review of Charles Bonnet hallucinations in psychiatry[16] illustrated in Table 7.1.

The checklist may also be used in longitudinal case series outcome studies, such as Gesundheit et al.'s[17] case series report (presentation and follow-up) of nine patients suffering from thyrotropin-secreting pituitary adenoma. Table 7.2 summarizes their findings and approach. This study was also performed according to a pre-established research protocol that is not always present in case series reports.

In contrast to single case reports that are mainly inductive, case series reports are a form of deductive research. Questions and hypotheses are formulated beforehand and the case series review is carried out to answer specific questions and to test hypotheses.

7.3.2.2 Case series with or without denominators

In toxicology, surveillance of unique cases is often used to better understand the toxic effects of various substances. For example, the increasing and often unjustifiable popularity of unconventional therapies has also produced new risks in the form of seemingly 'natural' and hence 'innocuous' treatments that are supposed to do only good. Anderson et al.[18] studied the toxicity of pennyroyal, a

Table 7.1 Evidence table of clinical case series in psychiatry: 13 cases of Charles Bonnet hallucinations

	SYSTEMATIC LISTING OF PATIENT CHARACTERISTICS*						OUTCOME*
Age	Sex	Cognitive impairment	Visual impairment	Living alone	Content of hallucinations	Insight	Cognitive state after one year
82	Female	Minimal	Severe	Yes	Two cats, five kittens	No	Unknown
73	Female	Mild dementia	Mild	No	Strangers (children)	No	Unknown
78	Female	Mild dementia	None	No	Landlord and family	No	Unknown
77	Female	Minimal	Mild	Yes	Strangers (young men)	No	Unknown
82	Female	Minimal	Severe	Yes	Strangers (children and adults)	Yes	Severe, rapid decline
71	Female	Mild dementia	None	Yes	Strangers (adults)	No	Unknown
84	Male	Minimal	Moderate	Yes	Strangers (adults)	Partial	Unknown
84	Female	None	Mild	Yes	Strangers (children and adults)	No	Severe, rapid decline
71	Male	None	Mild	No	Strangers (men)	No	Severe, rapid decline
75	Female	Mild dementia	Moderate	Yes	Strangers (adults)	No	Unknown
72	Female	None	Mild	No	Animals, human faces	Yes	Unchanged
80	Female	Mild dementia	None	Yes	Strangers (adults)	No	Unknown
70	Female	None	None	Yes	One cat	Yes	Unchanged

Source: Reference 16 – Reproduced with permission.
*Didactic additions.

Table 7.2 Outline of an evidence table of a case series in medicine. Abridged from a full review of nine cases of TSH-secreting pituitary adenomas

Case no.	Patient Age*	Sex	Initial diagnosis	Initial therapies	Date of diagnosis of TSH adenoma	Associated endocrine abnormalities	Subsequent therapies and operative findings	Results after therapies
1	51	M	Hypogonadism (1969)	Androgens,[131] Ithionamides Graves' disease	1982	Increased LH increased FSH	Pituitary surgery: invasive macroadenoma; radiation	Persistent tumour monocular blindness
3	43	F	Nonfunctioning pituitary tumour (1956)	Transfrontal hypophysectomy (1956) Radiation (1956)	1983	Increased growth hormone, clinical acromegaly	Pituitary surgery: invasive macroadenoma	Death
5	35	F	Graves' disease (1976)	Thionamides[131]	1983	Increased prolactin	Pituitary surgery: invasive macroadenoma	Persistent tumour
9	40	M	Graves' disease (1980)	Thionamides, subtotal thyroidectomy	1986	Increased prolactin	Pituitary surgery: invasive microadenoma	Biochemical normalization

Source: Reference 17 – Reproduced with permission.
*Age at time of diagnosis of TSH adenoma. TSH = thyroid-stimulating hormone; LH = luteinizing hormone; FSH = follicle-stimulating hormone.

herbal abortifacient with potentially lethal hepatotoxic effects, available in some health food stores.

Four cases observed longitudinally by other authors and eighteen previous case reports provided information about the toxicity of this herbal medicine, known since Roman times. The objective of this case series study was to better understand the toxicity of the substance rather than to study the occurrence of exposure and intoxication in a well-defined target population as denominator.

In other situations, denominators are available. Braun and Ellenberg[19] provide a descriptive epidemiology of adverse effects of immunizations per population of 100,000 in the United States. Their case series involved 38,787 adverse effect cases.

7.3.2.3   Case series from a single source

Case series originating from a single source such as one hospital, department, laboratory etc. have two obvious advantages: first, the experience with multiple cases usually elicits more direct questions and second, hypotheses and their study may be carried out deductively. Gesundheit *et al.*'s[17] mainly qualitative study of clinical and paraclinical features of thyrotropin-secreting pituitary adenomas falls into this category.

Other studies, however, highlight a particular team's experience, such as D'Abrigeon *et al.*'s[20] observation of five cases of papillomatosis of the biliary tract (papillary adenoma or papillary adenocarcinoma).

A predetermined protocol is highly desirable. For example, Braun *et al.*'s[21] study of snowmobiling-related brachial plexus injuries was based on a systematic retrieval of socio-demographic and behavioural characteristics of injured individuals, injury accident characteristics, diagnostic methods, associated injuries, signs and symptoms of brachial plexus involvement, and follow-up data, when available.

The enormous advantage offered by case series from a single source is the possibility of selecting and describing cases according to uniform clinimetric criteria of case detection, diagnosis, selection, measurement of selected variables, and final categorization and interpretation.

A systematic description of cases should lead to their synthesis as a basis for new hypotheses and more justified indications for the practice concerned. Dennis et al.[22] found a higher than expected number of elderly patients suffering from systemic lupus erythematosus with associated psychiatric problems such as confusional states, dementia and depression. A more common occurrence of this problem in the elderly as well as diagnostic criteria and strategies of detection were hypothesized.

Singh and Scheld[5] used their cases of rhabdomyolysis to research the infectious compared with the non-infectious aetiology of this clinical entity.

7.3.2.4 Case series from the literature

Sometimes, casuists are limited in their studies to case series found in the literature. In these situations, the authors may identify their own and rare observations first, for example a malignant intracerebral nerve sheath tumour[23], a pulmonary blastoma[24] or a cytomegalovirus pericarditis[25]. Such first personal observations form the index case, to which records and reports from the literature can be linked.

Case series constituted in such a way have a major disadvantage with regard to the variable heterogeneity of definitions, measurement criteria, diagnostic and therapeutic strategies and decisions, and follow-ups. It is the authors' responsibility to indicate in their studies the value and limitations of their findings stemming from this type of problem inherent in case series assembled 'from the outside'.

7.3.3 Follow-up of outcome studies or longitudinal case series

7.3.3.1 Follow-up of observational case series

When there is more than one reported examination of patients, longitudinal studies are produced. In contrast, instant or 'snapshot' pictures of cases are based on one measurement and evaluation only.

Longitudinal studies, as repeated examinations of case series in time, focus on various disease outcomes. Survival, longevity, cure, remission, pain resolution, normal organ function, return to normal values of biological variables, resumption of everyday life activities, and social and professional reintegration of the patient are just some of the challenges of outcome research. Their particular application to dentistry by Anderson[26] is worthy of attention.

Broadly defined, an **outcome** can be *'any possible result that may stem from exposure to a causal factor, or from preventive and therapeutic interventions: all identified changes in health status arising as a consequence of the handling of a health problem'* [27].

Currently, many case reports and case series reports lack an *a priori* definition and a choice of outcome. Justification of a chosen outcome is rare, especially with regard to clinical decisions that have to be modified or made.

However, the number of outcome-focused case series is increasing. For example, Tiffany *et al.*[28] followed a series of patients with refractory arrest rhythms. In contrast to the contraindication of thrombolytic therapy in patients receiving cardiopulmonary resuscitation, the authors hypothesized that this intervention in selected patients might facilitate their outcome in terms of the spontaneous return of circulation.

Bloom *et al.*[29] carried out a prospective study of visual acuity in 147 AIDS patients with cytomegalovirus retinitis. These authors concluded that standard treatment for this condition minimizes loss of vision and might protect previously uninfected eyes.

Hence, outcome case series studies of one group of patients are similar in their basic organization (and they should be) to Phase I or early Phase II clinical trials that aim to establish how healthy (Phase I) or diseased (Phase II) individuals will respond to treatment[30]. (N.B. To complete the picture, let us remember what follows Phases I and II. Phase III is a randomized controlled clinical trial based on the comparison of two or more groups. Phase IV consists of trials without patient preselection, while Phase V is based on trials that include patients with various co-morbidities and co-treatments for the latter.)

If Phase I or II clinical trials require an adequate protocol, so too do longitudinal case series studies focusing on various outcomes. From the methodological point of view, the latter must be considered as early phases of clinical modalities evaluations by experimental means.

7.3.3.2   Follow-up of experimental case series

In an experimental design, the researcher must decide which patient will be treated and which treatment will be offered (a certain drug, placebo, nothing etc.).

Case series studies can also be organized from an experimental point of view. However, only alternative designs to classical randomized controlled clinical trials are possible for obvious reasons.

An A-B-A design was used by Papageorgiou and Wells[31] to study the effects of attention training on the improvement of affect, illness-related behaviour and cognition in hypochondriasis sufferers. Patients acted as their own control. 'A' was the treatment under study, while 'B' was the withdrawal of the treatment period. The results obtained suggested that hypochondriacs might also benefit from the therapy under study.

Inherent characteristics of case series studies, such as the reduced number of patients and their heterogeneous origins and the management of such studies, limit the conclusions that can be drawn from these studies. Nevertheless, although case series studies are often the only feasible option, this should not mean that case series studies can be incorrectly prepared and interpreted.

7.3.4 'Meta-analysis' or systematic reviews of cases and case series

In the past twenty years, an increasing number of researchers in psychology, education and the health sciences have felt the need to integrate independent findings from different sources and studies focusing on the same topic or research problem. In the field of quantitative research, an 'analysis of analyses' or **meta-analysis** has been defined, methodologically developed and used increasingly, especially in the area of experimental research and clinical trials.

In the health sciences, the first textbooks on meta-analysis[32,33] appeared about ten years ago. Since then, a rapid development of quantitative methodology in meta-analysis and a widening of its applications have positioned this type of systematic review of evidence well beyond the scope of these first works. However, occasional updates[34] are worthy of attention.

We have defined **meta-analysis in medicine and allied health sciences** as '*a systematic, organized and structured evaluation and synthesis of a problem of interest, based on the results of many independent studies of that problem (disease cause, treatment effect, diagnostic method, prognosis etc.). Results of different studies become a new unit of observation and the subject of study is a new cluster of data, similar to groups of subjects in original studies. It is a 'study of studies' or 'epidemiology of their results'. Its objectives are: to confirm information, to find errors, to search for additional findings (induction) and to find ideas for further research (deduction)*'[13,32,33]. Meta-analysis must have both qualitative and quantitative components[13,32,34].

By substituting individual case studies or case series reports as a unit of observation, is there a need for the **meta-analysis of cases and of case series reports**?

Just as the results of original studies are heterogeneous, so are those of clinical case reports and case series reports. Is there a way to integrate them to obtain the most accurate picture of the disease and its control, especially when only isolated case reports are available?

The idea is relatively new, but it is a logical evolution of thinking in qualitative and quantitative research. Simultaneously but independently, conceptual proposals have appeared in qualitative research[35-37] as well as in the first *'meta-analyses of case reports and case series reports'*[38-41].

Jensen and Allen[35] investigated wellness and illness based on 112 qualitative studies of individuals suffering from a wide variety of health problems. They called their synthesis and inductive interpretation 'meta-analysis'. Criteria for the selection of qualitative studies for aggregation were proposed at the same time by Estabrooks, Fields and Morse[36]. 'Interpretive meta-synthesis' was used later by the same Jensen and Allen[37] to describe this kind of endeavour. Independent of the terms selected, an attempt was made to outline a better method of preparing aggregate case reports.

In clinical oncology, Nayfield and Gorin[42] retrieved from the literature twenty-one cases of tamoxifen-related ocular toxicity in breast cancer sufferers: one cohort and five small cross-sectional studies of occurrence of ocular findings in tamoxifen recipients. Their review of these cases produced a clearer picture of the nature and distribution of the toxicity, as well as of the severity of the ocular findings, which is useful in the management of tamoxifen-treated patients. They recognized the difficulty of attributing ocular findings to tamoxifen and other competing causes of retinal, macular and corneal abnormalities.

Fraser, Grimes and Schultz[38] evaluated an 'overload' of antigen in expectant mothers which mimicked the presentation of fetal antigen during pregnancy as a therapy for recurrent spontaneous abortion. Two meta-analyses, one aggregation of case series findings and one of three clinical trials, both provided evidence against its use until future randomized controlled clinical trials proved otherwise.

Nordin[39] made a 20-year literature review of both case reports and case series reports of primary carcinoma of the fallopian tube. This author was able not only to outline more appropriate patient characteristics, but also to hypothesize on the underdiagnosing of cases, causes of treatment failure, lack of controlled trials and usefulness of a 'second look laparotomy' for monitoring disease response to the treatment given (extensive debulking surgery and adjuvant platinum-based combination chemotherapy).

Drenth *et al.*[40] retrieved from the literature 126 articles on erythermalgia. Nine children in the articles met the inclusion criteria for the meta-analysis of cases. Descriptive characteristics of patients, spectra of clinical management, and treatment results were quantified across this set of observations. It was found that erythromelalgia might be associated with elevated blood pressure. Prognosis and treatment effect across the cases seemed different in primary and secondary erythermalgia. However, conclusions were limited due to the nature of a single case group study retrieved from the literature.

Cook *et al.*[41] also reviewed both case series and case reports in studying the outcomes of traumatic optic neuropathy in patients classified according to the standardized grading system. Recovery was related to the severity of the initial injury.

Obviously, none of these meta-analyses of cases is explanatory. Only prevalent case characteristics and case outcomes can be better assessed at this level of clinical research.

Establishing prevalent characteristics or average or typical values of observations in cases is similar to establishing **typical odds ratios** or other summary characteristics in clinical trials or in aetiological observational research. Such a **quantitative meta-analysis** usually follows a **qualitative meta-analysis**, i.e. *'a method of assessment of the importance and relevance of medical information coming from several independent sources through (by) a general, systematic and uniform application of pre-established criteria of acceptability of original studies representing the body of knowledge of a given health problem or question'* [13,32,34].

This kind of assessment of original studies in meta-analysis also applies to the systematic review of cases. However, we should explore and develop such **qualitative meta-analysis of cases** before regrouping them by other means. Until now, this has not been attempted. Noone has explored the quality or the completeness of information from one case to another even though this would enable us to better understand if such a qualitative review of cases is possible and realistic or not. Should this be a requirement in the future? The answer is probably.

By comparing case integration to a remarkable set of meta-analyses of clinical trials, it can be seen that research synthesis of case reports and case series reports marks only the beginning. The future will show how far we can go in this area.

7.4 CONCLUSIONS

Anyone who searches for evidence of what is helpful or harmful to patients is not necessarily satisfied with conclusions drawn from case reports and case series reports[43,44]. But if no other more adequate evidence is available, the best of this first line of evidence must be taken into account.

If this line of evidence is limited, and it often is, this is not a justification to reject it. On the contrary, it is a justification to use the evidence as well as possible within its own limits in a generally descriptive observational study.

Califf[45] states: '. . .*Case series without a control group will remain interesting because of the intrinsic importance of observation in medicine. Although individual case reports should never be taken as definitive evidence that practice should be changed, the importance of astute, appropriate bedside observation cannot be overestimated'*.

If an 'astute clinical observation' is at the root of case reports, should we teach young clinicians 'astuteness' and, if so, how should this be done?

Let us also realize that clinical case reporting is the clinician's most frequent exposure to medical research. The vast majority of practitioners will never carry out cohort or case control studies or complex clinical trials. Nevertheless, they should be as proficient clinical case reporters as possible.

The hierarchy of evidence proposed and adopted in North America[45-47] places descriptive studies at a very low level:

The strongest:	I	Randomized clinical controlled trials (at least one).
	II – 1	Well-designed non-randomized controlled trials.
	II – 2	Well-designed cohort or case control studies (preferably multicenter).
	II – 3	Multiple time series or place comparisons with or without interventions (including uncontrolled experiments, like at the onset of the antibiotic era).
The weakest:	III	Opinions of respected authorities, based on clinical experience, **descrip-**

tive **studies** or reports of expert committees.

Sackett's[43] levels of evidence show a similar structure:

The strongest:	Level I	Randomized trials carrying low alpha and beta errors.
	Level II	Randomized trials carrying high alpha and beta errors.
	Level III	Non-randomized concurrent co-hort comparisons (simultaneous observational comparisons of more than one group, e.g. treated and not treated subjects).
	Level IV	Non-randomized historical co-hort comparisons of more than one group, with control groups from the past originating either from the same institution or from the literature.
The weakest:	Level V	**Case series without controls.**

> Case reports and case series reports may be the 'lowest' or the 'weakest' level of evidence 'of a cause', but they often remain the 'first line of evidence of what happened'. This is where everything begins.

Let us note that such hierarchical classifications are not unequivocally accepted. Is a poorly designed randomized controlled clinical trial really better than an impeccable case control study? Does evidence from studies giving information about an 'average patient' apply to other patients, belonging to various diagnostic or prognostic subgroups? What should be done concerning decisions focusing on soft data or outcome measures that have not yet been evaluated by a soft data focused clinical trial (patient comfort, well-being etc.)[48]? What should be done if potentially adverse effects and undesirable outcomes from co-morbidities and their treatment are one of the main concerns?

All levels of evidence should be closely examined. How any level and hierarchy of evidence should be applied is the responsibility of its users.

Nevertheless, we can agree that in case series without controls *'the reader is simply informed about the fate of a group of patients. Such series may contain extremely useful information about clinical course and prognosis but can only hint at efficacy'* [43]. Obviously, the 'information' and the 'hint' should be as accurate as possible.

It is for this particular reason that case experience, case reports and case series reports must be as correctly carried out and presented as any other line of evidence. The *quality of data* and the *scope of interpretations and recommendations* are perhaps their most important assets. *The eligibility of record linkage of cases from independent sources* should also be respected. If cases originate from a one-source observation, they must be as sound methodologically as Phase II clinical trials.

If case reports and case series reports are of high quality, they really shouldn't be constrained by space limitations in medical journals. They do not deserve this fate. If space is excessively limited, the reader's only recourse is usually to hypothesize about the quality and completeness of the case report itself and its message. The 'underdogs of medical evidence' should be raised at least to the level of 'foot soldiers of evidence' who shoot as well as their guns let them.

Let us conclude on a lighter note. Was our historical example of the Immaculate Conception really a unique case report? Others[49] have assembled an impressive array of similar cases from diverse historical and religious contexts: Adonis, Zoroaster, Krishna, Mithra, Gautama Buddha, Dionysus, Quirmus, Attis and Indra. In fact, an evidence table could help identify known virgin mothers, including Maya (Gautama Buddha), Nama (Attis) and Devaki (Krishna), and the geographical location of such cases (Babylon, India, Tibet, Phrygia, Greece, Rome) would favour the occurrence of the event in question in the temperate climates of Asia or along the shores of the Mediterranean. Two additional births, those of Dionysus and Mithra, even took place in stables. (Incidentally, the latter was also born on December 25th.) Such an apparently more frequent occurrence than expected no doubt requires a more complete case series report, sources of data permitting, especially since the location of events in time suggests a sudden drop in the number of new cases in the past few centuries!

Our case series reports should be better and more complete.

REFERENCES

1. Coates M-M. Writing for publication: Case reports. *J Hum Lact*,1992; **8**(1): 23–6.
2. Instructions for authors. *Obstet Gynecol*,1994; **83**: six title pages (unnumbered).
3. Simpson RJ Jr, Griggs TR. Case reports and medical progress. *Persp Biol Med*,1985; **28**: 42–6.
4. Kamarulzaman A, Briggs RJS, Fabinyi G, Richards MJ. Skull osteomyelitis due to Salmonella species: Two case reports and review. *Clin Infect Dis*,1996; **22**: 638–41.
5. Singh U, Scheld WM. Infectious etiologies of rhabdomyolysis: Three case reports and review. *Clin Infect Dis*,1996; **22**: 642–9.
6. Jenicek M. Making clinical pictures or describing disease in an individual, pp. 125–136 in: *Epidemiology. The Logic of Modern Medicine*. Montreal: Epimed International, 1995.
7. Seltzer A. Multiple personality: A psychiatric misadventure. *Can J Psychiatry*, 1994; **39**: 442–5.
8. Huth EJ. The review and the case-series analysis, pp. 64–68 in: *How to Write and Publish Papers in the Medical Sciences*. Philadelphia: iSi Press, 1982.
9. Jenicek M. Picturing disease as an entity. Describing disease occurrence in the community, pp. 136–145 in: *Epidemiology. The Logic of Modern Medicine*. Montreal: Epimed International, 1995.
10. Grimes DA. Technology follies. The uncritical acceptance of medical innovation. *JAMA*,1993: **269**: 3030–3.
11. Milne R, Chambers L. Assessing the scientific quality of review articles. *J Epidemiol Comm Med*,1993; **47**: 169–70.
12. Hagell P, Odin P, Vinge E. Pregnancy in Parkinson's disease: A review of the literature and a case report. *Movement Disorders*,1998; **13**: 34–8.
13. Jenicek M. Meta-analysis in medicine: Where we are and where we want to go. *J Clin Epidemiol*,1989; **42**: 35–44.
14. Mulrow C, Oxman A. *How to Conduct a Cochrane Systematic Review*. San Antonio: San Antonio Cochrane Center, 1996.
15. The Potsdam International Consultation on Meta-Analysis. Potsdam, Germany, March 1994. Edited by WO Spitzer. *J Clin Epidemiol* (Special Issue), 1995; **48**: 1–171.
16. Cole MG. Charles Bonnet hallucinations: A case series. *Can J Psychiatry*,1992; **37**: 267–70.
17. Gesundheit N, Petrick P, Nissim M *et al*. Thyrotropin-secreting pituitary adenomas: Clinical and biochemical heterogeneity. Case reports and follow-up of nine patients. *Ann Intern Med*,1989; **111**: 827–35.

18. Anderson IB, Mullen WH, Meeker JE *et al*. Pennyroyal toxicity: Measurement of toxic metabolite levels in two cases and review of the literature. *Ann Intern Med*, 1996; **124**: 726–43.

19. Braun MM, Ellenberg SS. Descriptive epidemiology of adverse events after immunization: Reports to the Vaccine Adverse Event Reporting System (VAERS), 1991–1994. *J Pediatr*,1997; **131**: 529–35.

20. D'Abrigeon G, Blanc P, Bauret P, Diaz D, Durand L, Michel J, Larrey D. Diagnostic and therapeutic aspects of endoscopic retrograde cholangiography in papillomatosis of the bile ducts: analysis of five cases. *Gastrointest Endosc*,1997; **46**: 237–43.

21. Braun BL, Meyers B, Dulebohn SC, Eyer SD. Severe brachial plexus injury as a result of snowmobiling: a case series. *J Trauma Injury Infect Crit Care*,1998; **44**: 726–30.

22. Dennis MS, Byrne EJ, Hopkinson N, Bendall P. Neuropsychiatric systematic lupus erythermatosus in elderly people: a case series. *J Neurol Neurosurg Psychiatry*, 1992; **55**: 1157–61.

23. Sharma S, Abbott RI, Zagzag D. Malignant intracerebral nerve sheath tumor. A case report and review of the literature. *Cancer*,1998; **82**: 545–52.

24. Cutler GS, Michel RP, Yassa M, Langleben A. Pulmonary blastoma. Case report of a patient with a 7-year remission and review of chemotherapy experience in the world literature. *Cancer*,1998; **82**: 462–7.

25. Campbell PT, Li JS, Wall TC *et al*. Cytomegalovirus pericarditis: A case series and review of the literature. *Am J Med Sci*,1995; **309**(4): 229–43.

26. Anderson JD. The need for criteria reporting treatment outcomes. *J Prosthet Dent* 1998; **79**: 49–55.

27. *A Dictionary of Epidemiology*, 3rd Edition. Edited by JM Last. New York: Oxford University Press, 1995.

28. Tiffany PA, Schultz M, Stueven H. Bolus thrombolytic infusions during CPR for patients with refractory arrest rhythms: Outcome of a case series. *Ann Emerg Med* 1998; **31**: 124–6.

29. Bloom PA, Sandy CJ, Migdal CS, Stanbury R, Graham EM. Visual prognosis of AIDS patients with cytomegalovirus retinitis. *Eye*,1996; **9**: 697–702.

30. Jenicek M. Phases of evaluation of treatment, pp. 213–215 in: *Epidemiology. The Logic of Modern Medicine*. Montreal: Epimed International, 1995.

31. Papageorgiou C, Wells A. Effects of attention training on hypochondriasis: a brief case series. *Psychol Med*,1998; **28**: 193–200.

32. Jenicek M. *Méta-analyse en médecine. Évaluation et synthèse de l'information clinique et épidémiologique. (Meta-analysis in Medicine. Evaluation and Synthesis of clinical and epidemiological Information.)* St Hyacinthe and Paris: Edisem and Maloine, 1987.

33. Petitti DB. *Meta-analysis, Decision Analysis, and Cost-Effectiveness Analysis. Methods of Quantitative Synthesis in Medicine*. Monographs in Epidemiology and Biostatistics, Volume 24. New York and Oxford: Oxford University Press, 1994.

34. Jenicek M. Meta-analysis in medicine. Putting experiences together, pp. 267–95 in: *Epidemiology. The Logic of Modern Medicine*. Montreal: Epimed International, 1995.

35. Jensen LA, Allen MN. A synthesis of qualitative research on wellness–illness. *Qualit Health Res,*1994; **4**: 349–69.

36. Estabrooks CA, Filed PA, Morse JM. Aggregating qualitative findings: an approach to theory development. *Qualit Health Res,*1994; **4**: 503–11.

37. Jensen LA, Allen MN. Meta-synthesis of qualitative findings. *Qualit Health Res,*1996; **6**: 553–60.

38. Fraser EJ, Grimes DA, Schultz KF. Immunization as therapy for recurrent spontaneous abortion: A review and meta-analysis. *Obstet Gynecol*, 1993; **82**: 854–9.

39. Nordin AJ. Primary carcinoma of the fallopian tube: A 20-year literature review. *Obstet Gynecol Survey,*1994; **49**: 349–61.

40. Drenth JPH, Michiles JJ, Özsoylu S. Erythermalgia Multidisciplinary Study Group. Acute secondary erythermalgia and hypertension in children. *Eur J Pediatr,*1995; **154**: 882–5.

41. Cook MW, Levin LA, Joseph MP, Pinczover EF. Traumatic optic neuropathy. A meta-analysis. *Arch Otolaryngol Head Neck Surg,*1996; **122**: 389–92.

42. Nayfield SG, Gorin MB. Tamoxifen-associated eye disease: A review. *J Clin Oncol*, 1996; **14**: 1018–26.

43. Sackett DL. Rules of evidence and clinical recommendations. *Can J Cardiol,*1993; **9**: 487–9.

44. Peipert JF, Gifford DS, Boardman LA. Research design and methods of quantitative synthesis of medical evidence. *Obstet Gynecol,*1997; **90**: 473–8.

45. Califf RM. How should clinicians intepret clinical trials? *Cardiol Clinics*, 1995; **13**: 459–68.

46. Canadian Task Force on the Periodic Health Examination. *The Canadian Guide to Clinical Preventive Health Care*. Ottawa: Health Canada, 1994.

47. Preventive Services Task Force. *Guide to Clinical Preventive Services*, 2nd Edition. Baltimore: Williams & Wilkins, 1996.

48. Feinstein AR, Horwitz RI. Problems in the 'evidence' in 'evidence-based medicine'. *Am J Med,*1997; **103**: 529–35.

49. Knight C, Lomas R. *The Hiram Key*. London: Arrow Books Ltd, 1997.

Expanding
single case and
case series
research:
beyond simple
reports of
observations

CHAPTER 8

Expanding single case and case series research: beyond simple reports of observations

Reporting what has been seen and offering ideas on what might be done next is an extremely valuable experience in itself. However, more can be done on the basis of single cases or case series, since the methodology is already in place and experience increases the understanding of the depth and scope of the problems under study. In light of this, are case reports and case series reports still 'murky waters of evidence research'? Not quite.

Clinimetrically, an otherwise valid picture of a case is a good starting point for further observational research or for decision-oriented research based on a clinical trial. Let us consider these examples:

A **single case** serves as a sole research unit promoting better decision making related to treatment. The n-of-1 clinical trial, which is also called 'single patient trial' (SPT), was conceived with this purpose in mind.

Case series are often small and applicable only for particular research questions and studies. They are usually not 'statistically robust', although innovative research in genetic epidemiology has attempted to use them. Case–control studies with no controls were derived from this field.

8.1 SINGLE CASE RESEARCH: PATIENTS AS 'CASES'

Single case research has long been well rooted in two areas: psychiatry and nursing. Paying the utmost attention to the understanding and well-being of each and every patient is at the core of this approach. In fact, every single case subject to psychoanalysis can be considered a kind of applied qualitative research on a particular patient.

Health professionals in these and other fields aim to move beyond information about groups of patients. They want to adapt these findings or to contrast them with findings from a specific individual.

8.1.1 Historical roots of single case research in psychology, social sciences and mental health

As it often happens, medicine adopts, modifies, reorients, and expands principles, methods, and techniques from other fields of human endeavour. Sometimes, it is a distant connection such as with business or military arts (decision making); at other times, ideas and stimuli come from a closer neighbourhood, like psychology or social sciences. The latter contributed significantly to single subject research as we know it today. Kratochwill, Kazdin, Barlow and Hersen or Bromley's fundamental writings[1-4] give us a valuable insight and understanding of this domain.

Since the 1950s and 1960s, there has been a will to understand better and in more depth what happens in individuals, why it happens and with what results. Let us remember too, that 'statistically valid' observational and experimental research is not always possible because of technical, economical, ethical, political or societal reasons of feasibility.

A more solid methodological structure was given to studies of individuals. A periodic process of measurement of changes in an individual or series of individuals following experimental or non-experimental intervention was termed **time series**. Intervention periods (A) and subsequent periods of expected effect (B) or their multiples were structured in **AB** or **ABAB designs**. Following a similar search for consistency of cause–effect relationships in other health sciences, similar events were studied at different times and in different settings in a **multiple-baseline design** of research. An *ad hoc* statistical methodology followed as reviewed in the original monographs quoted above[1-4].

Classical single case research started 'statistically nude' with no sampling, no inferential statistics, no groups to study, no target populations (except the patient), no randomization, no stratification and no multivariate analysis. Instead, focus is on baseline assessment, quality of observation and recording of data or interpretation. Repeated measurements and replications are here to improve the quality of observation. Clinimetric rigour of definitions, eligibility criteria, quality and quantity of interventions and outcome measurements need to be implemented systematically.

In single case experimental designs, there is reliance on repeated observations over time[1]. As already mentioned above, the design is either before (A) and after (B) intervention or repeated over time such as in an **AB** and **ABAB** design (Figure 8.1).

Compulsive gambling or nail-biting treatments are given as examples applying to more serious mental and other health disorders[5].

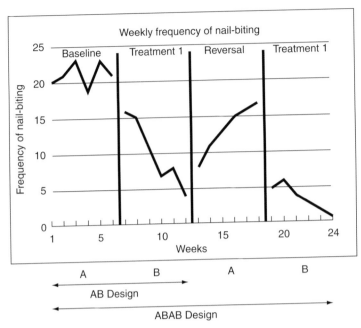

Figure 8.1 – AB and ABAB design in single case research in mental health. Source: Reference 5, reproduced with permission

Another design used is a **multiple baseline design**[5], as illustrated in Figure 8.2. Here, an AB design is repeated at different points in time. If such multiple AB comparisons lead to similar conclusions, the effectiveness of an intervention under study can be further investigated and a better confirmation of a potential cause–effect relationship can be reached.

8.1.2 'N-of-1' or 'single patient' trials

Physicians need answers to help them make the best possible therapeutic decisions. They may know from randomized controlled clinical trials that several drugs help treat a given disease. But to establish what works best for a specific patient, Guyatt *et al*[6,7] and others[8] have proposed the methodology of an '*n*-of-1' trial. Their remarkable ideas were based on a simple assumption that a single case research experience from a domain such as psychotherapy might be used with appropriate refinements and adaptation to drug treatment and other interventions in medicine. As a

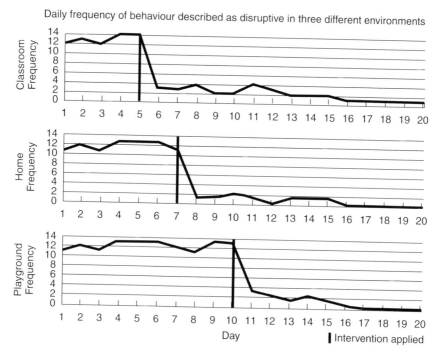

Daily frequency of behaviour described as disruptive in three different environments

Figure 8.2 – Multiple baseline design in a single case study. Source: Reference 5, reproduced with permission

clinical trial, they should remain as close as possible to the rules of randomized controlled clinical trials as we know them from clinical pharmacology and clinical epidemiology.

Here is how it works.

In any search for causes in epidemiology, comparisons are made by studying subjects exposed to a presumed cause of disease occurrence or its improvement and those not exposed to the factor under study. Figure 8.3 illustrates how these studies are organized[5].

The major difference between such an aetiological observational and experimental causal research is that the quality of evidence stemming from experimental research such as clinical trials is enhanced by a random assignment of patients in groups under study and two or more 'blindings': most often, physicians do not know what kind of treatment patients receive and patients do not know if they are receiving an active drug or a placebo. Results from such clinical trials help determine which treatment works best for

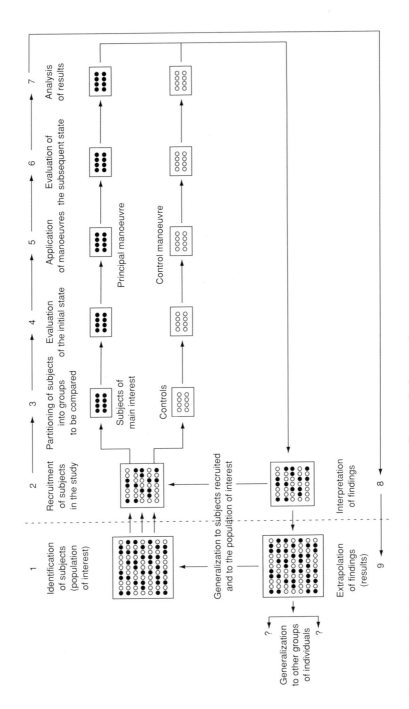

Figure 8.3 – Architecture of analytical studies. Source: Reference 9

patients having similar characteristics as those enrolled in a clinical trial and having a similar spectrum and gradient of disease.

But, in reality, what works best for Ms Jones who is sitting in my office? She suffers from headaches, and in clinical trials, several analgesics have proven useful. How can I know which one is most suitable for Ms Jones? What would be the best treatment for Mr Smith who suffers from asthma? And what specific treatment would most benefit Mr Miner who has chronic obstructive lung disease?

Having these kinds of questions in mind, several original papers introduced the n-of-1 clinical trials to medical readers, focusing on concepts[6,7], and more indepth methodological[10] and statistical[11-13] considerations and methods. An entire symposium[14] on single case studies tried to establish links between the past and present experience and to overview the new domain.

Many diseases are chronic, with protracted discomfort or without a frequently occurring episodic course: migraine, arthritis, tension headache, herpes, asthma, or gout. So why not try to randomize treatment of disease specifically in each individual concerned? Especially if treatments under consideration act fast and have short washout periods?[7] This is the novel idea behind a single patient trial: i.e. sample size, n, being 'one'. **Instead of randomizing patients (or treatments from one patient to another), alternative treatments are given at random for each forthcoming period of trial. Hence, treatments are randomized rather than patients.**

The n-of-1 clinical trial was designed specifically for chronic disorders and they have been successfully carried out in protracted problems such as asthma, chronic obstructive lung disease, vasovagal syncope, atopic dermatitis, Menière's disease, senescent forgetfulness, bulimia binges, chronic headache, fibrositis, stable angina, rheumatoid arthritis, irritable bowel syndrome, and Parkinson's disease.

Schematically, an 'n-of-1' trial in medicine is organized in such a way that, most often, an individual is a subject of a pair of treatment periods. These periods are well-defined and comparable in duration. During one period, which lasts often two or four weeks, the patient receives an active drug. (N.B. The duration of these periods may vary according to the nature of disease and its treatment.) During the other period of equal duration, he or she receives a placebo or any other active drug, subject to the patient's particular disease. The outcome measures may be an alleviation or disappearance of disease signs or symptoms, lesser occurrence of disease spells, or clinical cure.

The order of the two periods within each pair is randomized. Always in a random allocation, pairs of treatment periods are repeated, often three times or as often as required for the particular treatment preferred by the patient and his or her doctor. Also, as in any classical clinical trial, an *n*-of-1 trial may be stopped at any time for ethical reasons, patient's choice, overwhelming evidence, or other motive.

There are several ways in which to randomize. It may be done by tossing a coin, or as illustrated in Table 8.1. For example, a sequence of random numbers is taken from a computer-generated table of random numbers. The investigator decides that even numbers will identify the experimental treatment (A), and odd numbers (B) will mark the control treatment. Pairs of treatment periods, blinded if possible to the executioners and participants of the study, are applied in a sequence given by the table of random numbers.

Table 8.1 Sequence of treatments in an *n*-of-1 clinical trial. An example

Sequence of random numbers:	30702 52...	.....	.....	etc.
Sequence of first treatments in pairs of trial periods:	BABAA BA...	.....	.....	etc.
Experimental treatment: A Control treatment: B				

Randomization is described further in other sources[15]. Multiple blinding[9] is applied if feasible, as it is in a classical design of a clinical trial. Other related statistical considerations can be found in the literature[15].

This kind of crossover design can prove useful in cases[6]:

- where no randomized trial was conducted whatever the reason may be;
- when the health problem is rare;
- when the patient does not meet the criteria of eligibility for a classical randomized controlled clinical trial;
- perhaps most importantly, **when the decision must be specific to an individual patient;**
- when some patients would not benefit from a treatment option in a conventional clinical trial; and
- when a clinical trial came to negative conclusions about a given treatment, but some participants benefited from it.

As with any other kind of clinical research, an *n*-of-1 clinical trial must respect several criteria of its acceptability[7,8]:

- It must be **indicated** for the patient in terms of expected treatment effectiveness and patient's interest.
- It must be **feasible** in terms of
  - treatment quality, quantity and duration;
  - disease clinimetric characteristics (course, measurability);
  - ethics (duration, stoppability of treatment); and
  - in its specific practice setting.

The most important conclusion of an *n*-of-1 clinical trial is that it shows **what is best for a particular patient beyond the more general evidence.** The more general and less specific truth must be sought in conventional clinical and field trials. However, should we consider some kind of systematic integration and review of single patient trials[16]?

In a single patient trial, Wulff[17] recommends that clinical effect be measured by means of clinical scores and ranking methods and that statistical significance be measured using a permutation test. He also warns that the risk of Type II error is usually high in an *n*-of-1 trial.

The spectrum of applications of single patient trials is expanding. Some more recent examples can be found in medicine[18,19], surgery[20], psychiatry[21] and occupational medicine[22]. Other fields will certainly be added to the list to the benefit of individual patients.

An evaluation of several years of experience of many authors with *n*-of-1 trials appears positive[18, 22–24].

We may conclude that two major benefits arise from the *n*-of-1 clinical trials:

- Patients benefit from better fitting, 'made to measure' treatments.
- A scientific rigour from classical clinical experimental research is brought into single patient research, well beyond a simple uncontrolled observation, analysis and interpretation.

Currently, we may only speculate that proper integration of *n*-of-1 clinical trials in patients suffering from the same problem might complement results from classical clinical trials. The primary result of the latter is how the treatment works in one group if compared with the other. The former adds a 'personal fit'.

Developing and practising this domain further is well worth consideration, because the result of an *n*-of-1 clinical trial may be the best evidence – for Ms Jones, Mr Smith, or Mr Miner.

8.2 CASE SERIES RESEARCH: PATIENTS AS 'CASES'

Case series research is usually focused on the description of what has been seen in a set of cases one by one. However, more information can be obtained if we study extensively more than one case of disease.

Case series:

- can originate from a collection of cases as they come to the attention of a clinician;
- can be assembled retrospectively from existing medical records;
- can be assembled from various sites in a meta-analysis of cases, or a meta-analysis of case series themselves can be attempted.

8.2.1 Case–control studies 'with no controls'

It has jokingly been said that epidemiologists are 'eternally searching for suitable control groups'. There is some truth in this. When searching for some causal links, comparisons must take place. But what should be done if control groups are simply not available?

Genetic epidemiology has a suitable answer, at least for its own field.

Case series are somewhat like 'cases with no controls'.

But what is **genetic epidemiology**? It is defined as *'the science that deals with the aetiology, distribution and control of disease in groups of relatives, and with inherited causes of disease in populations. The study of the role of genetic factors and their interaction with environmental factors in the occurrence of disease in human populations ...'* [25]. It is an outgrowth of **molecular epidemiology**, *'... the use in epidemiological studies of techniques of molecular biology ...'* [25]. We have defined genetic epidemiology elsewhere as *'... the study of occurrence, causes and controllability of disease in relation to genetic factors ...'* [9] In both cases, some endogenous characteristic is studied as an independent variable (cause) related to the dependent one (health disorder). Other exogenous causal factors may be included in an expansion of this basic consideration.

While studying hereditary factors, geneticists usually find some clusters of index cases, which trigger a further search for the role of genetic or environmental factors [26]. Small-area studies of an excess of disease cases either do not follow a putative course, or look for a possible link with some environmental factors (carcinogenic substances in air or water) or hereditary factors (cancer families, ethnic or cultural groups).

Case studies where clusters are 'cases' should be properly analysed, explained and followed. Case series of patients also represent a database for cluster analysis. Therefore, how much more can be done with a single case series with no control group as a basis for comparison?

In a classical case–control study, two groups are usually assembled: a group of disease cases and a control group of those (healthy or suffering from another health problem) who do not have the disease. Once assembled, researchers examine, individual by individual, who was exposed to a factor of interest. Then, computing and looking at odds ratios and aetiological fractions, the researchers can estimate the strength and specificity of association [9]. Figure 8.4 illustrates such a directionality of a case–control study in comparison to the cohort. The investigator initially assembles a series of 'consequences' (cases) and 'non-consequences' (controls) and goes 'backwards' in identifying exposures in all the subjects under study. N.B. A cohort study works in the opposite direction by going from a 'cause' to its 'consequence'.

Are case–control studies without controls actually different? Yes and no. In 1990, Lehrer *et al*.[27] published a study of association of spontaneous abortion in women with breast cancer, a variant human oestrogen receptor gene and the wild type (B variant) gene. One single case series of breast cancer patients was assembled; their pregnancies and pregnancy outcomes were recorded as well as the gene occurrence in this patient group. Hence, one group of patients was 'split' into 'cases' (spontaneous abortions) and 'controls' (full-term pregnancies) and numbers of women carrying wild type or polymorph genes were identified (Figure 8.5).

This way, groups to compare were chosen from within a single case series and no controls exterior to the breast cancer cases were sought. But as we can see (Figure 8.5), there is a kind of a control group after all, although it is within the same set of patients. Mean number of spontaneous abortions was compared in women carrying different genes and a similar comparison was made for full-term pregnancies. The use of odds ratios and other measurements of association was developed only in more recent studies.

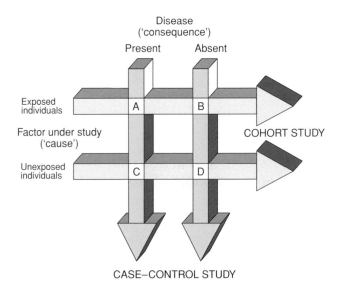

Figure 8.4 – Directionality of case–control and cohort studies. Source: Reference 9, reproduced with permission.

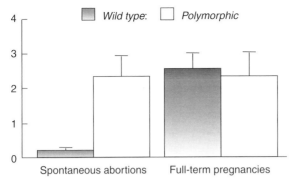

Mean (SE) number of spontaneous abortions per woman and mean (SE) number of full-term pregnancies per woman.

There was a significantly higher number of spontaneous abortions per woman in polymorphic women ($t' = 3.14$, df $= 7.32$, $p = 0.016$ by separate variance estimate), but the number of full-term pregnancies per woman was not significantly different ($t = 0.41$, df $= 29$, $p = 0.682$).

Figure 8.5 – Making subgroups within a single clinical case series while looking for an endogenous factor. Source: from Reference 27 reproduced with permission

The odds ratio derived from a single case series is usually represented by incident cases in the ratio of the relative risk for developing marker-positive disease to the relative risk for developing marker-negative disease[28]. As proposed by Khoury and Flanders[29] for the study of gene–environment interactions, differences between basic contingency tables in classical case–control and case series design can be seen in Table 8.2.

Note: Notation of categories in fourfold and other contingency tables as the example in Table 8.2 varies considerably across the medical literature. In classical cohort or case–control studies, a, b, c, and d are used either in horizontal or vertical order. Readers are warned that in this chapter, subjects representing categories in contingency tables of case–control studies with no controls are classified differently from other epidemiological studies: they are marked in this text as e to p. Reading of the literature should be made with these differences in mind.

Table 8.2 brings together three different designs for comparison. The first design is used in classical case–control studies studying exogenous (environmental) factors as possible causes of disease. The second design is used in gene–environment interaction analysis in the context of case–control study. Khoury and

Table 8.2 Design of a classical case–control study and a case–control study 'with no controls' in genetic epidemiology: Source: Adapted from reference 29

Classical case–control study of an environmental factor (2×2 design)	Classical case–control study for a gene-environment interaction analysis (2×4 design)	Case only study ('with no controls') for a gene–environment interaction analysis (2×2 design)

Classical case–control study of an environmental factor (2×2 design)

	Cases	Controls
Exposed (+)	a	b
Unexposed (−)	c	d

Odds ratio (OR) = ad/bc

TWO GROUPS

Classical case–control study for a gene-environment interaction analysis (2×4 design)

Exposure	Susceptibility genotype	Cases	Controls
−	−	e	f
−	+	g	h
+	−	i	j
+	+	k	l

OR genotype (OR_g) = fg/eh
OR exposure (OR_e) = fi/ej
OR genotype, exposure (OR_{ge}) = fk/el

Synergy index (SIM) = $OR_{ge}/OR_g \times OR_e$

TWO GROUPS

Case only study ('with no controls') for a gene–environment interaction analysis (2×2 design)

	Susceptibility genotype −	Susceptibility genotype +
Exposure −	m	n
Exposure +	o	p

Case only odds ratio (COR) = mp/no
COR = SIM

ONE GROUP

Flanders[29] propose to display data in a 2 × 4 table. In this design, unexposed subjects with no susceptibility genotype are used as a reference group to compute odds ratios for all other groups. Joint odds ratios (OR_{ge}) can be compared with odds ratios studying exposure alone (OR_e) and the genotype alone (OR_g). The third design is used to assess the magnitude of the association between exposure of interest and the susceptibility genotype. Case subjects are used only. A more detailed method of analysis of interaction between gene–environment factors based on this study design is beyond the scope of this book. It may be found in the more specialized epidemiological literature[27-34].

Researchers are often interested in identifying whether an effect under study is more than additive, i.e. if there is a synergy of exogenous and endogenous factors related to the health problem of interest. A **synergy index** (SIM) helps them decide if the joint action of these factors is multiplicative.

Another use of the case only method (Khoury – personal communication) may be considered in situations where two case groups that may have different possible aetiological factors serve for comparisons of subgroups with respect to exposures, genes or their combinations. Breast cancer with or without p53 mutations in the cancer tissue, trisomy 21 due to maternal origin vs. paternal origin errors may serve as examples of domains where such an approach might apply. In such situations, since there is no control group, this method detects the extent to which a risk factor is more important in one case group compared with the other. However, it may miss completely the situation when two cases groups have the same risk factors.

In summary, Andrieu and Goldstein[30] state that these associations are examined among cases only (diseased individuals) and offer an overview of available methods. The case–control with no controls study design follows the same epidemiological principles of case selection as any case–control study[30].

Advanced qualitative analytical methods were developed mostly in observational aetiological research[31,32], but Zhu[33] attempted a similar approach in the assessment of interventions in public health (telephone counselling in a community smoking cessation program). Casson et al.[34] brought this methodology into cancer surgery by studying the risk and prognostic factors and markers and survival in relation to p53 alterations (gene mutation and protein accumulation) in the case series follow-up of 61 surgically resected oesophageal cancers.

We can expect an even more expanded use of single case series aetiological and evaluative research in the near future.

8.3 OTHER DEVELOPMENTS

Recently, studies of cases have become increasingly influenced by two developments in medical research. On the one hand, the integration of results of independent studies has become a valuable tool creating an 'epidemiology' of study results[9,35-37] to improve decision making in medicine based on a wider volume of information than single studies separately. **Systematic reviews** of evidence are considered by some as a term qualifying **research integration** by adding evaluation of the quality of evidence to quantitative methods of integration as elaborated in **meta-analysis** at its origins.

On the other hand, a mutual respect is developing between protagonists of 'hard research' based on quantitative methods and techniques of epidemiology and biostatistics and innovators in 'soft research' in terms of **qualitative research** as already outlined in Chapter 2.

8.3.1 Cases and case series as subject to systematic reviews: meta-analysis of cases

As outlined in the previous chapter, research integration of cases is gaining in strength. It is therefore natural for investigators to try to do the most with the best available evidence, however limited it may be, by using simple cases and case series.

Single case reports can be assembled from a single source such as a hospital[37] or they can be brought together from different times and places[38]. This already proved useful a half a century ago to Wynder and Graham[39] whose case series indicated tobacco smoking as a potential aetiological factor in bronchial carcinoma followed by more advanced aetiological research. Elsewhere, simple observations of human behaviour in relation to full moon exposure[40] (full moon and madness) led to a creative explanation of biological plausibility as one of the criteria of causality in the health sciences. In another search for aetiology, intracranial neoplasms were studied in relation to the petrochemical research environment from which this case series originated[41]. Treatment effectiveness may be hypothesized first by studying case series such as those in the treatment of bipolar disorders in psychiatry[42].

Single case series may also be 'split' as genetic epidemiologists do, to allow research of associations other than on gene–environment interactions. Cook et al.[43] attempted this to study the effectiveness of treatment of traumatic optic neuropathy, labelling their study a 'meta-analysis' based on an assembly of multiple single cases experience. Success or failure of treatment, outcomes or other clinical events may be studied and hypothesized according to patient clinical characteristics within a single case series[44-46].

Case series are also being integrated in various specialties. In the oncological field, Robinson et al.[47] performed a meta-analysis of case series from various single institutions to analyze erectile functioning of men treated either by surgery or radiation for prostate carcinoma. In surgery, Shea *et al.*[48] brought together various case series from the literature to get a better understanding of mortality and complications associated with laparoscopic cholecystectomy.

Scientifically speaking, **hypothesis generation** is the main benefit of this kind of study.

The methodology of such a **meta-analysis of cases and case series** will certainly be further refined in the near future.

8.3.2 Case studies as qualitative methodology in health services research: situations as 'cases'

Traditionally, health services studies relied on quantitative research. Recently, a qualitative approach through case studies was discussed in the literature[49].

For example, the problem of overcrowding in hospital emergency departments was examined. Based on quantitative research, patient demographic and clinical characteristics were identified and patients were counted. Waiting time, number of emergency personnel attending, bed availability and other factors were also counted, tabulated and analysed and conclusions drawn. This problem could be analysed based on qualitative methods which focus on a more detailed understanding of what is happening, namely, patient decisions and motivations for use of services, interaction between the patients and their family, ambulance crews, medical personnel at the hospital, hospital administration reasoning values and other elements which at the beginning may be hard to define, obtain and quantify.

Qualitative research helps clarify values, language and meanings attributed to individuals involved in both sides of an emergency services overcrowding problem: the consumers and providers. Subjects are encouraged to speak freely rather than responding to prepared data sheet of questions.

In quantitative research, outcomes are defined in advance. In qualitative research, the full range of desired and undesired outcomes is not known in advance and at the outset[49]. For these authors, qualitative research helps further the understanding of many questions in our example:

- How did those implementing emergency services perceive the intentions of their planners?

- Did both have the same agendas? If not, what were the agendas?
- Was the original plan implemented or not? Why?
- What were the difficulties in running the service?
- What problems were solved and unsolved?
- What changes were made, which ones were not and why?

Qualitative research findings help focus more clearly on quantitative research in order to develop messages and materials in social campaigns and educational interventions[50].

Unstructured observations and interviews, long-term work in a given setting, detailed inquiries by the investigator who becomes a part of the setting and process under study, are part of a qualitative inquiry.

The qualitative approach is recommended when the level of uncertainty is high, theory and direction obscure, and situations are novel and complex[49].

Case reports based on individuals such as clinical case reports and **case reports based on situations and their settings** may be combined. A situation as a case may be the closing of a hospital, the opening of a chronic care facility, or the new organization and functioning of pre-hospital emergency services in trauma and cardiopulmonary arrest resuscitation or symptom relief.

Also, qualitative and quantitative findings may be linked to reach a better understanding and to find more acceptable solutions to the problem.

For example, a clinician wishes to get a better understanding of pain in his or her patients. In his/her inquiry, the distinctions between qualitative and quantitative research are rather blurred. Based on a quantitative approach as in clinimetrics, he/she will try to characterize pain in terms of duration, frequency of spells, intensity, etc. In his/her qualitative study, the clinician will attempt to grasp his/her patient's circumstances, values or perception of pain. This could apply to nausea in cancer patients, vertigo in neurology or anxiety in psychiatry.

Elsewhere, the clinical approach may be inductive and qualitative. When a psychiatrist asks his patient, 'What's on your mind? What do you think about it? How do you feel about it?' he performs a kind of qualitative research.

The **study of cases** is thought of slightly differently in qualitative research: causation is not seen through the epidemiological comparison and analysis of risk characteristics, but it is understood conjecturally[51].

Qualitative researchers identify case–control (retrospective) studies as the *study of necessary causes* or *case-oriented research* and cohort studies (prospective) are considered *studies of sufficiency* or *variable-oriented research*. The researchers complain, perhaps rightly so, that associations under study are defined in advance as a restrictive way of pre-setting and defining dependent and independent variables[51].

Using multiple sources for collecting evidence is called *triangulation*. All six sources of evidence have their own strengths and weaknesses: documentation, archival records, interviews, direct observations, participant-observation and physical artefacts. From such a *source of information linkage* should arise a kind of *case study database* analogous to the laboratory or field research[52].

Contemporary qualitative studies require a research protocol as rigorous as for observational analytical studies or clinical trials in clinical and fundamental epidemiology. Their publication is now evaluated as thoroughly as the quantitative research reports[53].

The results should be based on good internal (credibility) and external (transferability) validity, reliability (dependability) and objectivity (confirmability) as in quantitative research. The necessary attributes of qualitative research are also close to 'mainstream' research: values and objectives guiding the research, research question, context, study design – sampling – data collection and analysis, strategies and techniques for enhancing rigor, presentation of findings[53].

Strategies to enhance the rigor of qualitative research from all these angles are proposed in the literature[54].

8.4 CONCLUSIONS

All the diversification and improvements in qualitative research methodology and its interface with quantitative research will only enhance Califf's conclusions about case and case series reports[55]: '. . . *although individual case reports should never have been taken as a definitive evidence that clinical practice* (and health services management) *should be changed, the importance of astute* bedside (and field) *observation cannot be underestimated ... case series without a control group will remain interesting because of the intrinsic importance of observation in medicine. ...'*

A widening spectrum of relevant methodology and an array of 'cases', individuals or situations, lead to innovative approaches linking quantitative and qualitative thinking, research and decision in medicine and other health sciences.

Medicine can only benefit from such important lessons drawn from anthropology, sociology or nursing experience. The terms used may be different at times, but common and complementary thinking are here to stay.

REFERENCES

1. *Single Subject Research. Strategies for Evaluating Change.* Edited by TR Kratochwill. New York: Academic Press, 1978.
2. Kazdin AE. *Single-Case Research Designs. Methods for Clinical and Applied Settings.* New York and Oxford: Oxford University Press, 1982.
3. Barlow DH, Hersen M. *Single Case Experimental Designs. Strategies for Studying Behavior Change,* 2nd Edition. New York: Pergamon Press, 1984.
4. Bromley DB. *The Case-Study Method in Psychology and Related Disciplines.* Chichester and New York: John Wiley & Sons, 1986.
5. Ricketts T. Single case research in mental health. *Nurs Times,*1998; **94**(23) Jun10–16: 52–5.
6. Guyatt G, Sackett D, Taylor WD, Chong J, Roberts R., Pughsley S. Determining optimal therapy – randomized trials in individual patients. *N Engl J Med,*1986; **314**: 689–92.
7. Guyatt G, Sackett D, Adachi J, Roberts R, Chong J, Rosenbloom D, Keller J. A clinician's guide for conducting randomized trials in individual patients. *CMAJ,*1988; **139**: 497–503.
8. N-of-1 trials: selecting the optimal treatment with a randomized trial in an individual patient. Pp. 173–5 in: Sackett DL, Scott Richardson W, Rosenberg W, Haynes RB. *Evidence-Based Medicine. How to Practice and Teach EBM,* 2nd Edition. New York and Edinburgh: Churchill Livingstone,1997.
9. Jenicek M. *Epidemiology. The Logic of Modern Medicine.* Montreal: EPIMED International, 1995.
10. Guyatt GH, Heyting A, Jaeschke R, Keller J, Adachi JD, Roberts RS. N of 1 randomized trials for investigating new drugs. *Contr Clin Trials,*1990; **11**: 88–100.
11. Sandvik L. Single case studies from a statistician's point of view. *Scand J Gastroenterol,* 1988; Suppl.147; **28**: 38–9.

12. Spiegelhalter DJ. Statistical issues in studies of individual response. *Scand J Gastroenterol*,1988; Suppl.147; **28**: 40–5.

13. Rochon J. A statistical model for 'N-of-1' study. *J Clin Epidemiol*,1990; **43**: 499–508.

14. *Single Case Studies*. Proceedings from a Symposium in Oslo, March 14–15,1987. Edited by H Petersen. *Scand J Gastroenterol*, 1988; Suppl.147,**28**: 1–8.

15. *Statistics in Practice*. (Gore SM, Altman DG). Articles from the British Medical Journal. London: British Medical Association,1982.

16. O'Brien PC. The use and misuse of N-of-one studies. *Int J Oral Maxillofac Impl*, 1997; **12**: 293.

17. Wulff HR. Single case studies. An introduction. *Scand J Gastroenterol*, 1988; Suppl.147; **28**: 7–10.

18. Guyatt GH, Keller JL, Jaeschke R, Rosenbloom D, Adachi JD, Newhouse MT. The *n*-of-1 randomized controlled trial: clinical usefulness. Our three-year experience. *Ann Intern Med*,1990; **112**: 293–9.

19. Mahon J, Laupacis A, Donner A, Wood T. Randomized study of *n*-of-1 trials versus standard practice. *BMJ*,1996; **312**: 1069–74.

20. McLeod RS, Cohen Z, Taylor DW, Cullen JB. Single-patient randomised clinical trial. Use in determining optimum treatment for patient with inflammation of Kock continent ileostomy reservoir. *Lancet*,1986; **1**: 726–8.

21. Marazzi MA, Markham KM, Kinzie J, Luby ED. Binge eating disorder : response to naltrexone. *Int J Obesity*,1995; **19**: 143–5.

22. Hodgson M. N-of-one clinical trials. The practice of environmental and occupational medicine. *JOM*,1993; **35**: 375–80.

23. Jaeschke R, Adachi J, Guyatt G, Keller J, Wong B. Clinical usefulness of amitriptyline in fibromyalgia: The results of 23 N-of-1 randomized controlled trials. *J Rheumatol*,1991; **18**: 447–51.

24. Larson EB, Ellsworth AJ, Oas J. Randomized clinical trials in single patients during a 2–year period. *JAMA*,1993; **270**: 2708–12.

25. *A Dictionary of Epidemiology*, 3rd Edition. Edited by JM Last. New York: Oxford University Press, 1995.

26. *Geographical and Environmental Epidemiology. Methods for Small-Area Studies.* Edited by P Elliot , J Cuzick, D English, R Stern. Published on Behalf of WHO Regional Office for Europe. Oxford: Oxford University Press, 1992.

27. Lehrer S, Sanchez M, Song HK, *et al*. Oestrogen receptor B-region polymorphism and spontaneous abortion in women with breast cancer. *Lancet*,1990; **335**: 622–4.

28. Begg CB, Zhang Z-f. Statistical analysis of molecular epidemiology studies employing case-series. *Cancer Epidemiol Biomarkers Prev*,1994; **3**: 173–5.

29. Khoury MJ, Flanders WD. Non-traditional epidemiologic approaches in the analysis of gene–environment interaction: Case–control studies with no controls. *Am J Epidemiol*,1996; **144**: 207–13.

30. Andrieu N, Goldstein AM. Epidemiologic and genetic approaches in the study of gene–environment interaction: an overview of available methods. *Epidemiol Rev*,1998; **20**: 137–46.

31. Piegorsch WW, Weinberg CR, Taylor JA. Non-hierarchical logistic models and case-only designs for assessing susceptibility in population-based case–control studies. *Stat Med,*1994; **13**: 153–62.

32. Umbach DM, Weinberg CR. Designing and analysing case–control studies to exploit independence of genotype and exposure. *Stat Med,*1997; **16**: 1731–43.

33. Zhu S-H. A method to obtain a randomized control group where it seems impossible. A case study in program e valuation. *Evaluation Rev,*1999; **23**: 363–77.

34. Casson AG, Tammemagi M, Eskandarian S, Reston M, McLaughlin J, Ozcelik H. p53 alterations in oesophageal cancer: association with clinicopathological features, risk factors, and survival. *J Clin Pathol: Mol Pathol,*1998; **51**: 71–9.

35. Jenicek M. *Méta-analyse en médecine. Évaluation et synthèse de l'information clinique et épidémiologique. (Meta-analysis in Medicine. Evaluation and Synthesis of Clinical and Epidemiological Information).* St Hyacinthe and Paris: EDISEM and Maloine,1987.

36. Jenicek M. Meta-analysis in medicine. Where we are and where we want to go. *J Clin Epidemiol,*1989; **42**: 35–44.

37. Williams M, Simms HH. Abdominal compartment syndrome: case reports implications for management in critically ill patients. *Ann Surg,*1997; **63**: 555–8.

38. Voulgarelis M, Dafni UG, Isenberg DA, Moutsopoulos HM. Malignant lymphoma in primary Sjogren's syndrome: a multicenter, retrospective, clinical study by the European Concerted Action on Sjögren's Syndrome. *Arthritis Rheum,*1999; **42**: 1765–72.

39. Wynder EL, Graham EA. Tobacco smoking as a possible etiologic factor in bronchiogenic carcinoma. A study of six hundred and eighty-four proved cases. *JAMA,*1950; **143**: 329–36.

40. Raison CL, Klein HM, Steckler M. The moon and madness reconsidered. *J Affect Disord,*1999; **53**: 99–106.

41. Delzell E, Beall C, Rodu B, Lees PS, Breysse PN, Cole P. Case-series investigation of intracranial neoplasms at a petrochemical research facility. *Am J Ind Med,*1999; **36**: 450–8.

42. Suppes T, Brown ES, McElroy SL *et al.* Lamotrigine for the treatment of bipolar disorder: a clinical case series. *J Affect Disord,*1999; **53**: 95–8.

43. Cook MW, Levin LA, Joseph MP, Pinczower EF. Traumatic optic neuropathy. A meta-analysis. *Arch Otolaryngol Head Neck Surg,* 1996; **122**: 389–92.

44. Merren MD. Gabapentin for treatment of pain and tremor: A large case series. *Southern Med J,*1998; **91**: 739–44.

45. Cohen DM Flament M, Dubos PF, Basquin M. Case series: catatonic syndrome in young people. *J Am Acad Child Adolesc Psychiatry,*1999; **38**: 1040–6.

46. Fisher H. A new approach to emergency department therapy of migraine headache with intravenous haloperidol: a case series. *J Emerg Med,*1995; **13**: 119–22.

47. Robinson JW, Dufour MS, Fung TS. Erectile functioning of men treated for prostate carcinoma. *Cancer,*1997; **79**: 538–44.

48. Shea JA, Healey MJ, Berlin JA *et al.* Mortality and complications associated with laparoscopic cholecystectomy. A meta-analysis. *Ann Surg,*1996; **224**: 609–20.

49. *Qualitative Methods in Health Services Research.* Edited by KJ Devers, S Sofaer, TG Rundall. *HSR (Health Serv Res),*1999; **34**: No.5, Part II–special issue.

50. Sofaer S. Qualitative methods: What are they and why use them? Pp. 1101–18 in Ref. 40.

51. Ragin CC. The distinctiveness of case-oriented research. Pp. 1137–51 in Ref 40.

52. Yin RK. Enhancing the quality of case studies in health services research. Pp. 1209–24.

53. Papers that go beyond numbers (qualitative research). Pp. 131–134 in: Greenhalgh T, Donald A. *Evidence Based Health Care Workbook. For Individual and Group Training.* London: BMJ Books, 2000.

54. Devers KJ. How will we know 'good' qualitative research when we see it? Beginning the dialogue in health services research. Pp. 1153–88 in Ref. 40.

55. Califf RM. How should clinicians interpret clinical trials? *Cardiol Clin,* 1995; **13**: 459–68.

CHAPTER 9

What next?

CHAPTER 9

What next?

Foretelling the future of clinical case reports is like making their prognosis. This prognosis is now more promising than ever, given the advances in casuistics made possible by clinimetrics and epidemiological thinking in clinical medicine and by the awareness that state of the art clinical case reports open Pandora's box and Croesus' trove of further medical research and knowledge

In the past ten years, the field of medical casuistics has been significantly refined and restructured. The spontaneity and compulsiveness of many casuists who used to provide information simply because they felt that they should, have been abandoned in favour of a more rigorous approach.

9.1 HOW CLINICAL CASE REPORTS SHOULD BE EXAMINED TODAY

The most important new paradigm of clinical case reports is the view that they open the gate to further more refined and more complete research. Clinical case reports are also a part of an increasing equilibrium between qualitative and quantitative research. Predominantly quantitative research usually follows case reports.

Most of us, to a certain degree, have been trained in epidemiology and have some knowledge of it as the basis for quantitative research and logic in medicine. Nevertheless, we may feel uncertain about recent methodological developments in qualitative research, especially from areas other than the health sciences. We also experienced those same feelings when meta-analysis was introduced, and when even the basic paradigm of medicine shifted from a deterministic view to a probabilistic view of the health phenomena that surround us. This is all now fading away.

Clinical case reports are competing for the attention of readers and for space in medical journals. The reports must now be as good as any other type of medical information and research.

The reader's occasional rapid loss of interest in reading a clinical case report can be attributed to several problems:

- Editors of medical journals who do not give authors enough information concerning what is expected of them and their work.
- Authors who do not have the knowledge required to determine the relevance and originality of their case(s), and to present their case(s) properly.
- Readers of clinical case reports who do not know how to draw relevant information from the case reports and how to judge the information's usefulness for their practice and research.

In other words, authors must know why the case should be reported and how to report it, editors must be explicit with regards to the publishing requirements of the case, and readers should be trained to properly interpret the message of a case report.

If a case report or a case series report is not clear enough in terms of:

- the reason for its presentation;
- its clinimetric explicitness;
- its explanation of facts and actions;
- its recommendations for practice and research stemming from the case(s) experience;

then the reader will remain perplexed, blasé and disinterested.

Clinical case reports also offer an invaluable additional asset. If they are prepared in a structured and organized manner, their authors learn how to organize and structure their own thoughts and practice. Hence, the clinical report is an important teaching tool[1–3], both for the author and the reader.

In public health and field epidemiology, case reports based on index cases 'of something bigger' remain powerful generators of hypotheses in the search for causes of outbreaks, epidemicity or pandemicity of disease, or in considering the need to evaluate the efficacy and effectiveness of health programmes.

Theoretically speaking, the outbreak of an epidemic is a 'situation', i.e. a 'case', with respect to the qualitative research outlined in Chapters 3 and 5. Handling and reporting a disease outbreak is therefore a 'case study' with additional important quantitative components. Its methodological rules go well beyond the scope of this reading and have been discussed in other sources[4].

Clinical research usually requires that a study deals with a considerable number of patients in order for it to be 'statistically powerful' and to minimize beta errors. Does this mean that case reports are 'powerless'? The answer is yes and no. In reality, they are undeniably strong since they lead to further observational, aetiological and experimental research. One situation should not exclude the other[5,6].

Cases are 'uncontrolled experiments'. They do not provide proofs, but they generate hypotheses. It is impossible to underestimate them for this latter reason. It should also not be forgotten that Darwin's and Freud's theories were founded on case observations, studies and reports and not on what we would today call 'serious aetiological and experimental research'[6].

Maple syrup disease was explained on the basis of first case observations and reports of progressive neurological degeneration and peculiarly odoriferous urine. These reports led to the hypothesis of a genetic error of metabolism, which was later confirmed[7].

Early reporting of important life- and health-threatening clinical cases also allows rapid emergency control measures to be put in place. Although aetiological confirmations follow later, at times some decisions simply can't wait. By way of example, one only has to think of the congenital malformations that occurred after thalidomide use[8].

Moreover, cases can lead to a future aggregation with other cases in either observational or quasi-experimental research. They should therefore be well defined in order to serve this purpose. Clinical microbiologists, toxicologists and psychiatrists often depend on them.

9.2 SUGGESTIONS TO ASPIRING CASUISTS

Accumulated from one generation to the next, the wealth of experience contained in clinical case reporting will continue to increase with time. To improve these reports even further, recently borrowed concepts from the areas of epidemiological thinking and methodological refinements in clinimetrics must be mastered and put to good use. These concepts are reflected in the following 'Ten Commandments':

- Persevere.
- Look for something new and relevant, worthy of sharing.
- Learn, adopt and use clinimetrics[9–11]. Observe and describe thoroughly. Correctly record what you have heard, seen, touched, smelt and read.

- Reason in terms of epidemiology.
- Temper your interpretations.
- Avoid exaggerated conclusions.
- Consider recommendations that stem from and are proportional to the experience of the case study.
- Retain only what is relevant for medicine and beneficial for the patient.
- Consider case series studies as rigorous descriptive studies of diagnosis, follow-up or prognosis without *a priori* statistical considerations. However, work up their design and protocol according to the rules and standards of Phase II clinical trials[12-16].
- While remaining critical, have fun, and be proud of your accomplishments. You are doing first rate clinical research within the limitations of clinical case reports.

Good clinical case reports are challenging. Often, there are no *a priori* hypotheses of disease aetiology. In addition, there is usually no *a priori* knowledge of the disease itself or of its course and control.

When several cases are regrouped, some heterogeneity is unavoidable. These cases are often detected haphazardly and are observed for different reasons, in different ways. Then, they are subjected to a 'boot camp' of case series research, where the final result expected is 'a nice line of uniformed soldiers marching in time and in line' toward a common purpose and goal. The endpoint of such a march should not signify the scientific death of the cohort we assembled in our hearts and minds.

9.3 WHAT REMAINS TO BE DONE

Most of the challenges of medical casuistics are related to its direction and methodology:

- Is it possible to define criteria more completely according to which case should be reported?
- Should we give a different form and structure to case reports, focusing on different problems such as challenging differential diagnosis, clinical management of an unexpected course and outcome or choosing between competing therapeutic and disease management plans?
- Should we make clinicians' and general practitioners' training in medical casuistics and proper clinical case reporting more formal and structured?
- If a clinical case report triggers expected further clinical research, is it logical and necessary to compare results from initial case observations and their interpretation with what is obtained at other stages in the research of the same problem?
- Would it be useful to refine and restructure specific presentation rules for series of cases?

The future will most likely provide answers to most of these questions. In the meantime, if this reading helps make health professionals more aware of the advances and challenges of today's medical casuistics, its objectives will have been met.

9.4   LET US CONCLUDE

Clinical case studies and reports are an inherent and indispensable part of medical research, progress and experience. Moreover, they are also very helpful in maintaining the human aspect of medicine and medical research. Despite knowing all about the numerical facts, probabilities, risks and chances relevant to them, patients will continue to ask their physicians: 'and what about me?' A 50 per cent case fatality rate may be a fact, but the patient is either dead or alive. In other words, a case remains a case, and a patient a patient, whether in practice or research.

Medical casuists must handle each case as a unique experience and as a broader part of medical knowledge, experience and generalized wisdom. The challenge is to manage both parts of the equation equally well.

As long as medicine exists, physicians will monitor John Doe or Jane Smith's pulse rate and blood pressure. They will also know the pulse rate and blood pressure levels in John and Jane's community. John and Jane are not at all interested in what is happening around them, but they want their blood pressure to be under control in order to avoid any life-threatening complications. Physicians will and must always make distinctions between individual cases and observations and generalizations arising from the study of many cases and individuals[17]. As they focus their decisions on individual cases, they must also aim to control the disease in the community. They must therefore use community experience to treat individual patients. Both approaches, patient- and community-centred, are complementary and necessary.

Is medical casuistics a science? Reiser[18] states that *'the classification of facts, and the recognition of their sequence and relative significance is the function of science'* as well as *'the habit of forming judgement upon these facts unbiased by personal feeling'*. In this light, and this is where the challenge lies, medical casuistics should be a part of the science of medicine.

Is the clinical case report only the first line of evidence in the formal aetiologic research in medicine? It may be more than that.

In 1975, Carol Buck[19] emphasized how hypothetico-deductive reasoning is important for epidemiologists. Thus she confirms Karl Popper's and Thomas Kuhn's philosophy of research. These philosophers of science consider a contradictory finding to be an important 'falsifier' or an overthrow of a current paradigm (*Gestalt switch*).

For Velanovich[20], 'the case report is relatively strong evidence that an existing paradigm is wrong if it provides evidence that does not corroborate the paradigm. However, it is relatively weak evidence for a new hypothesis even though it may be highly corroborative, because of fallacies in judgment associated with the law of small numbers, representativeness, and availability. In some very special cases, the information obtained from a case report may be the impetus for a "Gestalt switch" in a paradigm of medical and surgical thinking'.

Clinical case research remains an important element in maintaining an equilibrium between research based on solid numerical data and research based on individual clinical experience. This is a case of and for 'medical research and practice with a human face'.

Obviously, appropriate measurements, quantifications and categorizations help in individual cases here, as much as in cases beyond the field of medicine, such as human or animal 'beauty' contests. The rewards are either a crown or a clean bill of health.

If the reader still doubts that medical casuistics is a serious endeavour, he should raise his hand and be counted. After that, he should explain his reasoning!

REFERENCES

1. Loschen EL. The resident conference: A method to enhance academic intensity. *J Med Educ,*1980; **55**: 209–10.
2. Petrusa ER, Weiss GB. Writing case reports. An educationally valuable experience for house officers. *J Med Educ,*1982; **57**: 415–7.
3. Winter R. Edit a staff round. *Br Med J,*1991; **303**: 1258–9.
4. Jenicek M. Investigations of disease outbreaks, pp. 189–192 in: *Epidemiology. The Logic of Modern Medicine.* Montreal: Epimed International, 1995.
5. Feinstein AR. An additional basic science for clinical medicine: I. The constraining fundamental paradigms. *Ann Intern Med,*1983; **99**: 393–7.
6. Herman J. Experiment and observation. *Lancet,*1994; **344**: 1209–11.
7. Simpson RJ Jr, Griggs TR. Case reports and medical progress. *Persp Biol Med,*1985; **28**: 402–6.
8. Levine M, Walter S, Lee H, Haines T, Holbrook A, Moyer V for the Evidence-Based Medicine Working Group. Users' guides to the medical literature. IV. How to use an article about harm. *JAMA,*1994; **271**: 1615–9.
9. Feinstein AR. *Clinimetrics.* New Haven and London: Yale University Press, 1987.
10. Feinstein AR. An additional basic science for clinical medicine. IV. The development of clinimetrics. *Ann Intern Med,*1983; **99**: 843–8.
11. Jenicek M. Identifying cases of disease. Clinimetrics and diagnosis, pp. 79–118 in: *Epidemiology. The Logic of Modern Medicine.* Montreal: Epimed International, 1995.
12. Jenicek M. Phases of evaluation of treatment, pp. 213–215 in: *Epidemiology. The Logic of Modern Medicine.* Montreal: Epimed International, 1995.
13. Neiss ES, Boyd TA. Pharmogenology: The industrial new drug development process, pp. 1–32 in: *The Clinical Research Process in the Pharmaceutical Industry.* Edited by GM Matoren. New York and Basel: Marcel Drekker Inc., 1984.
14. Tannock I, Warr D. Non-randomized clinical trials of cancer chemotherapy: Phase II or III? *JNCI,*1988; **80**: 800–1.

15. The Protocol Review Committee, The Data Center, The Research and Treatment Division and The New Drug Development Office. Phase II trials in the EORTC. *Eur J Cancer,*1997; **33**: 1361–3.
16. Shoemaker D, Burke G, Dorr A, Temple R, Friedman MA. A regulatory perspective, pp. 193–201 in: *Quality of Life Assessments in Clinical Trials.* Edited by B. Spilker. New York: Raven Press, 1990.
17. Rose G. Sick individuals and sick populations. *Int J Epidemiol,*1985; **14**: 32–8.
18. Reiser SJ. Humanism and fact-finding in medicine. *N Engl J Med,*1978; **229**: 950–3.
19. Buck C. Popper's philosophy for epidemiologists. *Int J Epidemiol,* 1975; **4**: 159–68.
20. Velanovich V. The function of the case report in medical epistemology. *Theor Surg,* 1992; **7**: 91–4.

A LAYMAN'S GLOSSARY

Absolute risk reduction (ARR):
The absolute arithmetical difference in bad event rates for treated and untreated subjects in clinical trials or observational analytical studies. Synonym of *attributable risk* or *risk difference*. May also be expressed as an *absolute benefit increase*.

But for **cause (in law):**
The event that, but for its existence, another event would not have occurred. Also called a *sine qua non* cause.

Case (in general):
An individual, a given situation, an occurrence or an event in a particular area of daily or professional life.

Case (in medicine):
A particular instance of disease, as in *a case of leukaemia*. Sometimes used incorrectly to designate the patient with the disease. In this book, a patient has a specific case of a given health problem.

Case–control study with no controls:
A method developed in genetic epidemiology, to evaluate gene–environment interaction in disease aetiology. Case subjects only are used to assess the magnitude of the association between the exposure of interest and the susceptibility genotype. Analysis of contingency tables built within a single case series in the study of exposure and susceptibility genotype.

Case only study:	See *Case–control study with no controls.*
Case fatality (rate):	The proportion of cases of patients with a specified condition who die of it within a specified time.
Case report (clinical):	A structured form of scientific and professional communication normally focused on an unusual single event (patient or clinical situation). The case report aims to provide a better understanding of a case and of its effects on improved clinical decision making. A summary of a case study.
Case report in law and occupational health:	A clinical or public health case report focusing on a specific cause–effect relationship about the health condition of the case (patient) and environmental and medical factors potentially affecting the well-being of the patient, his/her peers or his/her personal and community environment. It is expected that the reporter will specify and demonstrate with satisfaction that the situation under study and the general experience corroborate and apply specifically to the case under litigation.
Case study:	A detailed description and analysis of an individual case which explains the dynamics, pathology, management and/or outcome of a given disease.
Case series study:	A detailed description and analysis of a series of cases which explains the dynamics, pathology, management and/or outcome of a

given disease. In *epidemiological terms*, it refers to the study of several individuals without denominators.

Casuist (in medicine): A practitioner of the study of clinical cases.

Casuistics (in philosophy): The application of general laws and rules to a particular area or fact. A method of solving problems by implementing actual actions based on the general principles and study of similar cases.

Casuistics (in medicine): The recording and study of cases of any disease. The observation, analysis and interpretation of clinical cases. The art of choosing, gathering, structuring and conveying pragmatic information about relevant clinical cases. Casuistics aims to provide a better understanding of a given health problem and therefore to improve clinical decisions.

Casuistry (in philosophy and theology): A system of rules for distinguishing right from wrong in everyday situations, usually associated with a concept of morality that views correct behaviour in terms of obedience to a set of closely defined laws. For some, it implies specious reasoning based on an excessive amount of minute, often unimportant detail. For hospital ethicists, it refers to the art of applying abstract principles, paradigms and analogies to particular cases.

Clinical data:	Clinical observations as seen, measured and recorded. Example: blood pressure 120/80 mmHg.
Clinical information:	The interpretation and meaning given to clinical data. Example: a normo-tensive patient.
Clinimetrics:	A field focused on indexes, rating scales and other expressions used to describe and measure symptoms, physical signs and other distinctly clinical phenomena in clinical medicine. A process extending from the retrieval of clinical observations to their description, interpretation, classification and categorization.
Collective case study:	See *Case series study.*
Co-morbidity:	All other health problems present in a patient studied and treated for a disease of interest. Example: diabetes or hypertension in a patient studied and treated for cancer.
Conceptual criteria or definitions:	The qualitative characterizations of phenomena under study. Example: a hypertensive patient under study.
Corpuscularianism:	A way of reasoning in law while considering a cause–effect relationship. Characterization of causation as collisions that follow the physical laws defined by mathematics. Derived from Newtonian physics portraying causation as a matter of mechanical contacts or collisions between particulate objects. Emphasizing deductive reasoning and mechanistic causal chain interpretations, more tradi-

tional in courts, positivism–corpuscularianism competes with probabilistic reasoning and uncertainty in epidemiology and medical reasoning today.

Criterion: A principle or standard by which something is judged. An element that serves as a basis for comparison (standard). Rules according to which observations are selected, measured, classified and interpreted. The term is used in the same way for recruitment of cases.

Cross-sectional study: A study based on a single observation and evaluation of cases. A *'single shot' study*, based on one examination of patients only. Synonym of *transversal study*.

Deductive research: Research based on the verification of the acceptability of *a priori* formulated hypotheses. Refers to research or studies that are built specifically to accept or refute a given question.

Evidence: Any data or information whether solid or weak, obtained through experience, observational research or experimental work (trials), which is relevant either to the understanding of the problem or the clinical decisions made about the case.

Evidence-based clinical case report: A case report focused on a defined question and its solution based on the evaluation of all relevant evidence available for the solution of the case.

Evidence-based health care: A discipline centred upon evidence-based decision making about individual patients, groups of patients or populations, which may be manifested as evidence-based purchasing or evidence-based management.

Evidence-based health service: Health care decisions focused on research-based evidence about the consequences of treatment augmented by the intelligent use of wider information about, for example, finance, patient flows and health care politics.

Evidence-based medicine: The process of systematically finding, assessing and using contemporaneous research results as the basis for clinical decisions. (Always look for the best available information and use it!) The application of simple rules of science and common sense to determine the validity of the information. The application of valid information to answer the clinical question. Patient care based on evidence derived from the best available ('gold standard') studies.

Evidence table: In meta-analysis, a *systematic* tabular compilation of the present and absent characteristics of original studies. In clinical case series studies, a similar compilation and review of case, time and place characteristics.

Genetic epidemiology: The science which deals with the aetiology, distribution and control of disease in groups of relatives, and with inherited causes of disease in populations. The study of the role of genetic factors and their interaction with environmental factors in the occurrence of disease in human populations. The study of occurrence, causes and controllability of disease in relation to genetic factors.

Gradient of the disease: The directional expression of the severity of a disease, similar to colour shades from light to dark, i.e. from unapparent to fatal cases of a disease.

Hard data: Clinical and paraclinical data that can be precisely defined and measured. Examples: heart rate, blood cell count.

Hardening of soft data: All means used to improve the criteria, measurement and quantification of soft data in order for the quality of soft data to match that of hard data as closely as possible.

Hermeneutics: A philosophical concept of interpretation and understanding; making sense of a mess of clinical and paraclinical data and information in a case. Derived from Hermes, the messenger of the gods in Greek mythology.

Hypothesis: A proposal or question that research or study should accept or refute.

Idiographic analysis: An analysis that is exclusive (or limited) to the case under study.

Idiographic approach (in philosophy): The advancement of science based on the information or what was acquired as information from one individual case.

Inception moment: Any moment at which the follow-up of a case begins: beginning of a clinical stage of disease, date of admission, etc. Must always be defined.

Incidence: The number of *new* events occurring in a given population in a defined period of time. For a more refined definition, see the epidemiological literature.

Index case: The first case in a family or other defined group (disease sufferers, etc.) to come to the attention of the investigator. Often used to formulate preliminary hypotheses and define criteria for selection and follow-up of cases to come, as in the investigation of an infectious disease outbreak. In medical genetics, an index case represents an original patient (propositus or proband) who provides the stimulus to study other members of the family in order to ascertain a possible genetic factor in causation of the presenting condition.

Inductive research: Research that proceeds from observations serving as a basis for hypotheses and answers. (Hypotheses are a product of the data that precedes them. Studies that originate data are not necessarily built to verify hypotheses and questions of interest.)

Initial state: The state of the patient (case) before clinical actions of interest (manoeuvres) are applied.

Instrumental case study:	A study focusing on a better understanding of the *problem* represented by the case.
Intrinsic case study:	A study focusing on a better understanding of the *case itself.*
Longitudinal study:	The follow-up of cases in time based on more than one examination. A *'burst of shots' study.* Synonym of *cohort study.*
Manoeuvre:	A clinical action under study, i.e. diagnostic procedure, surgical treatment, medical treatment or care etc.
Meta-analysis:	A systematic, organized and structured evaluation and synthesis of a problem of interest based on the results of many independent studies of that problem (disease cause, occurrence, treatment effect, diagnostic method, prognosis etc.). Epidemiology of the results of independent studies of the same problem of interest. A study of studies. A similar precise integration of cases in case series studies becomes a *meta-analysis of cases.*
Molecular epidemiology:	The use of molecular biology techniques in epidemiological studies.
Monographic study:	A study as detailed and complete as possible.
Multiple baseline design:	Study of similar events at different times and/or different settings in search of consistency of cause–effect relationships.
Narrative-based medicine	Process of obtaining qualitative information from the patient, which is used in subsequently improved clinical decision making.

n-of-1 research or trial: Any research on a single patient. In *clinical epidemiology*, it is a variation of a randomized controlled trial in which a sequence of alternative treatment regimens is randomly assigned to a patient.

Nomothetic approach (in philosophy): The advancement of science based on the information or on what was acquired as information from a set of cases.

Number needed to harm (NNT): Analogous to number needed to treat (NNT), i.e. the reciprocal of the difference in adverse effect rates. Number of patients who, if treated experimentally, would lead to one additional person being harmed compared with patients who received the control treatment.

Number needed to treat (NNT): The number of patients who need to be treated to achieve one additional favourable outcome. It is calculated as 1/absolute risk reduction.t

Occurrence study: Any study of frequency of disease or other attribute or event in a population. Usually a descriptive observational study of the prevalence, incidence, mortality or case fatality of a disease or of the prevailing characteristics of the individuals, time or place where a phenomenon of interest 'occurs'.

Operational criteria: Measurable rules of selection of cases and variables. Example: the cases to follow will be subjects with a blood pressure of 160/120 mmHg or higher than either of these values.

Outcome:	Any possible result that may stem from exposure to a causal factor, or from preventive and therapeutic interventions. All identified changes in health status arising as a consequence of the handling of a health problem.
Paradigm:	Any pattern or example. The way we look at things, events and actions around us.
Phase I clinical trial:	Clinical trial whose objective is to determine how *healthy individuals* will respond to the treatment (pharmacodynamics, tolerance, metabolism, adverse effects).
Phase II clinical trial:	Clinical trials whose objective is to determine how the disease *sufferer* will respond to treatment. Either one group of patients (early Phase II) or two or more groups (without *a priori* defined statistical considerations) are studied (late Phase II).
Phase III clinical trial:	A randomized controlled clinical trial. Subjects are randomly divided into at least two groups to be compared. Several factors are not revealed to the patients and investigators, such as the group to which the patients belong and the true outcome measured.
Phase IV clinical trial:	Similar to Phase III but without preselected patients. The patients enter the trial 'as they come through the door'. 'Clean' or 'neat' cases participate.
Phase V clinical trial:	In this situation, non-selected patients who suffer from various co-morbidities (diseases other than the one under study) and

Phenomenology: are treated for these additional health problems (co-treatments are present) participate in post-marketing studies.

The philosophical concept of research on the meaning of the experience lived by a case.

Prevalence: Cases existing at a given moment of study or observation. A more refined concept of prevalence is available in the epidemiological literature.

Prognosis: An assessment of the patient's future, based on probabilistic considerations of various beneficial and detrimental clinical outcomes as causally or otherwise determined by various clinical factors and biological and social characteristics of the patient and of the pathology (disease source) itself.

Prognostic characteristics: Characteristics of patients, a time or a place related to a particular probability of events in individuals *who already have the disease under study*. A common term for prognostic factors and prognostic markers (see below).

Prognostic factors: *Modifiable* patient, time or place characteristics related to the outcome of the health problem under study. Example: antibiotic treatment for infection.

Prognostic markers: *Non-modifiable* patient, time or place characteristics related to the outcome of the health problem under study. Example: age in degenerative joint diseases.

Qualitative meta-analysis: A systematic overview of characteristics and components of original studies of the same problem. A method of assessing the importance and relevance of medical information through a general, systematic and uniform application of pre-established criteria of acceptability of original studies representing the body of knowledge of a given health problem or question. A systematic assessment of the completeness and quality of the characteristics of cases represents a *qualitative meta-analysis of cases*.

Qualitative research: Any kind of research that produces findings not arrived at by means of statistical procedures or other means of quantification. Some data may be quantified but the analysis itself is a qualitative one. An in-depth study of unique observations.

Quantitative meta-analysis: The general, systematic and uniform evaluation and integration of *dimensions*, i.e. numerical findings, from independent studies of the same problem of interest. 'Typical' values for sets of studies are of primary interest. Examples: typical odds ratios, protective efficacy rates, etc.

Quantitative research: Research based on series of observations, where phenomena are measured, quantified, counted, described and analysed by statistical methods. An in-depth study of multiple observations.

Rate:	An expression of the frequency at which an event occurs in a defined population. The number of events (numerator) is related to all individuals that take part in them (denominator). More refined definitions are available in the epidemiological literature.
Relative risk reduction (RRR):	The proportional reduction in rates of bad events between control and experimental participants in a trial. Synonym of *aetiologic fraction, attributable fraction, attributable risk per cent, protective efficacy rate*. May also be expressed as a *relative benefit increase*.
Risk:	The probability that an event (disease, complication, improvement, etc.) will occur.
Risk characteristics:	A common term for risk factors and risk markers (see below).
Risk factor:	Any *modifiable* characteristic of persons, times or places related to disease occurrence. Example: smoking as a trigger of lung cancer.
Risk marker:	Any *non-modifiable* characteristic of persons, times or places related to disease occurrence. Example: age in relation to cancer or cardiovascular diseases.
Routine case report:	Structured oral or written communication of the experience with a clinical case within a defined space–time period, such as admission and discharge of the patient. Admission reports, progress reports, discharge summaries or experiences with cases

outside the hospital environment fall into this category. Their objective is the inter- and intra-professional continuity of communication, administrative needs and requirements. Also protection of the well-being of the patient himself and his entourage.

SOAP: Often, the first abbreviation that is learnt by any house officer writing patients' daily progress reports: **S**ubjective perception of the patient, **O**bjective data, **A**ssessment, and **P**lan of management of the case.

Soft data: Clinical and paraclinical observations that are difficult to define, measure and classify. Examples: sorrow, anxiety, paraesthesia.

Spectrum of the disease: The variability of the clinical picture in terms of the extent of the disease; similar to a spectrum or rainbow of colours. Example: all the systemic manifestations of infectious diseases.

Subsequent state: The state of the patient (case) following the clinical management (actions, manoeuvres) under study. It may or may not be the result of this management.

Theory: An interrelated set of constructs (variables) formed into propositions or hypotheses that specify the relationship among variables.

Time series: A periodic process of measurement changes in an individual or series of individuals following experimental or non-experimental intervention.

REFERENCES

1. *Dorland's Illustrated Medical Dictionary,* 24th Edition. Philadelphia and London: WB Saunders, 1965.
2. *Miller-Keane Encyclopedia and Dictionary of Medicine, Nursing and Allied Health,* 6th Edition. Philadelphia: WB Saunders, 1997.
3. *A Dictionary of Epidemiology,* 3rd Edition. Edited by JM Last. New York, Oxford and Toronto: Oxford University Press, 1995.
4. *New Illustrated Webster's Dictionary Including Thesaurus of Synonyms and Antonyms.* New York: Pamco Publishing Company, Inc., 1992.
5. Jenicek M. *Epidemiology. The Logic of Modern Medicine.* Montreal: Epimed International, 1995.
6. Related references quoted in the text of this book.

INDEX

Page numbers printed in **bold** type refer to figures and tables; those in *italic* relate to entries in the glossary.

without controls 162, 163, 164
cross-sectional descriptions 152
with/without denominators 152–5
description 148–9
and descriptive studies 148, 149,
    162–3
evidence tables 152, **153–4**, *212*
experimental, follow up 158
forms of 149
from literature 156
meta-analysis of cases 150, 158–61
number of cases included in 148
numerator focus 148
observational, follow up 156–7
outcome-focused 157
presentation of 151
reviewing several cases 152
from a single source 155–6
systematic reviews 150, 158–61
from a team's experience 155
case series reports
    data quality 164
    as first line of evidence 163
    interpretations, scope of 164
    linkage of cases from independent
        sources 164
    literature reviews 151
    methodological aspects 150–61
    in paediatric surgery **31**
    recommendations, scope of 164
    types of 151
    see also case reports
case series research 172, 180–5
    fields of application 186–7
case series studies **56**, *208–9*
    A-B-A design 158
    classification 149–50
    cross-sectional studies 150
    in epidemiology *209*
    longitudinal studies 150, 156–7, 158
    meta-analysis of cases 150
    numerator focus 148
    objectives 148
    see also multiple cases
case studies 52–3, **56**, *208*
    in administration, management,
        economics and business 49–50
    in biology 53
    collective 53
    concepts and design 49
    differential diagnosis 117
    empiric 50
    experimental 50, 53
    as first link in evidence chain 56–8

in human sciences 53
instrumental 53, *215*
intrinsic 52, *215*
in medical research 56–8
and medical training 58–60
meta-analysis of cases *see* meta-
    analysis
monographic 53, *215*
overview 49
qualitative and quantitative 50–1, 52
settings for 49
in social sciences 50–3
see also case series studies; multiple
    cases
'a case to learn from' 97
cases
    beginning of 109
    concept of case 51–2
    definitions 51–2, *207*
    end-point of 112
    as first line of evidence xviii
    in general *207*
    in medicine *207*
    multiple 7, 53, 60
    patients as *see under* patients
    relevance of 98–9
    situations as 55, 60, 60–1, 187–9
    stages of 105–6, **107**
    as uncontrolled experiments
        199–200
casuistics 45–6
    in daily life 48
    definitions 46
    direction of inference in 47, **48**
    in general understanding 48
    in medicine *see* medical casuistics
    origin of term 46
    in philosophy *209*
    as a research method 46
casuistry
    definitions 46, 47
    historical perspective 46–8
    in philosophy, theology and ethics
        46–7, *209*
casuists
    classical *vs.* clinical 99
    definitions 46, 46–7
    in medicine *209*
    modern 47
    suggestions to 200–1
causality criteria 86
causation, in law 84
cause–effect relationship
    in epidemiology 85–6

cause–effect relationship (cont)
  in occupational medicine 81–2
  in tort litigation 85–6
causes, necessary, studies of 189
Charles Bonnet hallucinations 152, **153**
civil courts 84
claims 70, 80–7
  in occupational medicine see
    occupational medicine
  see also tort litigation
claims-based medicine 22
classical case reports 97
clinical case reporting see case
  reporting
clinical case reports see case reports
clinical case series see case series
clinical case studies see case studies
clinical data 111, **113**, 210
  selection and quality of 100
clinical decisions 106
clinical epidemiology 5, 8, 16, 18, 50–1
  evaluation in 105–6
  n-of-1 research/trials 216
  reliance on xvi
  see also epidemiology
clinical experience viii, 21
clinical gradient see gradient of the
  disease
clinical information 100, **113**, 210
clinical spectrum see spectrum of the
  disease
clinical trials **56**
  phases I-V 157–8, 217
clinimetric criteria **113–15**
clinimetric indexes 110–11
clinimetrics
  in case series studies 149
  in clinical case reports 58, 105, **113–15**
  creation of 18
  definition 105, 210
  and qualitative research 89
  reliance on xvi
cluster analysis 181
CMAJ (Canadian Medical Association
  Journal) 7, 122, **124**
co-morbidity 111, **115**, 210
  in case report example 136
Cochrane Collaboration 29
cohort studies **56**, 57, 189, 215
  directionality 182, **182**
  see also longitudinal studies
collective case studies 53
  see also case series studies
colorectal cancer 77–8

compensation claims see claims; tort
  litigation
conceptual criteria/definitions 210
confidentiality 123
consequences 182
  webs of consequences and outcomes
    111
control groups **56**, 57
corpuscularianism 84, 210–11
course of disease 108–9, **114**
criminal courts 85
criterion 211
cross-sectional studies 150, 152, 211
cytomegalovirus retinitis in AIDS
  patients 157

data
  clinical data 100, 111, **113**, 210
  paraclinical data 111
  quality 100, 164
  soft and hard 100, **114**, 213
decision-making, role of EBM 25, 32–3
deductive reasoning in tort litigation
  84
deductive research 51, 211
dentistry, application of longitudinal
  studies 157
descriptive studies 148, 149, 162–3
  see also occurrence studies
deterministic medicine 4, 18, 27, 198
diagnosis, medical viii
  in case report example 139–40
Diagnostic and Statistical Manual
  (DSM IV) 74–5
diagnostic procedures 111
differential diagnosis 117
  in case report example 137, 140
discharge reports/summaries 70, 80,
  220
disease
  course of 108–9, **114**
  definition **113**
  disease spells 109–10
  gradient of 109, 110, **114**, 213
  induction period 109
  spectrum of 109, 110, **114**, 221
  see also occurrence studies
drugs see risk factors
DSM (Diagnostic and Statistical
  Manual) IV 74–5

EBM see evidence-based medicine
economics, case studies in 49–50
effectiveness of clinical practices 18, 76

efficaciousness of clinical practices 18,
  76
efficiency of clinical practices 18, 76
empiric case studies 50
epidemics, as situations 199
epidemiological research **56**
epidemiologists, hypothetico-
  deductive reasoning 203
epidemiology 50–1
  case series study *209*
  causality criteria 86
  cause–effect relationship 85–6
  genetic *see* genetic epidemiology
  molecular 19, 181, *215*
  shoe leather epidemiology 18
  of study 185
  see also clinical epidemiology
erythermalgia 160–1
erythroblastosis fetalis 99
erythromelalgia *see* erythermalgia
ethicists, in health care 47
ethics 123
  casuistry in 46–7, *209*
evidence
  best evidence 16, 19, 20–1, 21, 22
  characteristics 19
  definitions 18–19, *211*
  and experience 21
  hierarchy/levels of 162–4
  levels of 20
  low-level 20
  sources 17–18
evidence-based approach, specialties
  and fields in which applied 24–5
evidence-based case reports 32
evidence-based clinical case reports
  76–80, 119, *211*
  facets of 77
evidence-based conclusions 79
evidence-based discharge summaries
  80
evidence-based health care 22, *211–12*
evidence-based health service *212*
evidence-based medicine (EBM) xviii,
  21–33, **30**
  articles about 24
  challenge of 26
  clinical case reports in 15–42
  contrasts in concept of 28
  critiques 25
  decision-making role of 25, 32–3
  definitions **23**, *212*
  differing views about 25
  an evolving process 22–4

the future 29–30
goal **23**
historical context 17–18
journals 24
philosophy of 26–8
scope of 26
steps in **23**
evidence-based morning reports 77–8
evidence-based public health (EBPH)
  21, **30**
  definitions **23**
  goal **23**
  steps in **23**
evidence handling methodology 79
evidence tables 152, **153–4**, *212*
experience, clinical viii
  and evidence 21
experimental case series, follow-up of
  158
experimental case studies 50
experimental design, single case 53, 173
experimental research **56**

fallopian tube carcinoma 160
Flexner, Abraham 27
floor presentations 5

generalizations 53, 117
  vs. individual observations/cases 203
genetic epidemiology 19
  case control study with no controls
    207
  definitions 181, *212–13*
  study designs **184**
Gestalt switch 203
Glasgow Coma Scale 110
gradient of the disease 109, 110, **114**, *213*

hallucinations 152, **153**
hard data 100, **114**, *213*
  hardening of soft data 100, **114**, *213*
health service research, quantitative
  and qualitative 187–9
hermeneutics 105, *213*
hospital-focused case presentations 5,
  8, 95–6
hospitals, emergency department
  overcrowding 187
human sciences, case studies in 53
hypochondriasis 158
hypothesis *213*
hypothesis generation 61, 187, 199

idiographic analysis 117, *213*

idiographic approach 49
  in philosophy *213*
Immaculate Conception 58, 164–5
immunizations 155
inception moment *214*
incidence *214*
  see also occurrence studies
index cases 4, 17, 51, 56–7, 149
  definition 57, *214*
  examples 57, 58
  as generators of hypotheses 199
  in genetic studies 181
induction period, of disease 109
inductive research 51, 53, *214*
initial state 105, 106, 108, *214*
  in case report example 136–7
Injury Severity Score (ISS) 110
instrumental case studies 53, *215*
intensive designs 49
interpretive meta-synthesis 160
intra-subject-replication designs 49
intracranial neoplasms 186
intrinsic case studies 52, *215*
ISS (Injury Severity Score) 110

jargon, in case reports 122
Journal of Obstetrics and Gynecology 7
*Journal of the American Medical
  Association (JAMA)* 24, 102, 122
journals *see* medical journals
justification
  in case report example 139–40, 141
  of outcomes 157
  of single case reports 104

knowledge-based health service 22

laboratories, role of 16
The Lancet xi, 7, 97, 102
language, in case reports 122
laparoscopic cholecystectomy 187
law
  'but for' (*sine qua non*) cause 84, *207*
  case report in *208*
  causation 84
  proximate cause 84
literature reviews, in case series
  reports 151
litigation *see* claims; tort litigation
longitudinal studies 150, 156–7, 158, *215*
  see also cohort studies

madness, and the full moon 186
management, case studies in 49–50

manoeuvres 105, 106, *215*
  evaluation of **114**
maple syrup disease 200
medical casuistics 56–8
  challenges of 201–2
  definition 46, 59, *209*
  direction of inference in 47, **48**
  as entry link in evidence chain 56–8
  medical training and 58–60, 202
  method of handling cases 202–3
  published material 94–5
  as a science 203
  widened concept of 60
  see also case reporting
medical diagnosis viii
medical history, in case report example
  135–6
medical journals
  case reports in xi–xiii, 5, 6–7
  checklists 123
  editorial policies 6–7, 122
  evidence-based medicine articles
    and journals 24
  functions of xii
  guidelines for contributors 94, 96–7
  journals' expectations of case
    reports 94–5, 97–123, **124**
  readers' loss of interest in reports
    198–9
  see also case reports; publishing
medical research, steps in **56**, 57
medical training
  astuteness in observation 162
  by the bedside 59
  case presentation in 8
  case reports as teaching tools 8, 32,
    199
  in clinical case reporting 202
  in clinical case studies 58–60
  in medical casuistics 58–60, 202
  relationships in viii
  in study of individuals 6
medicine
  narrative-based 89, *215*
  routine clinical case reports in 70–1,
    76
Medline xii, 151
mental health, single case research in
  172–4
meta-analysis 51, 55, 160
  of cases 150, 158–61, *215*
  definition 21, 159, *215*
  qualitative 21, 159, 161, *218–19*
  quantitative 21, 159, 161, *219*

228   INDEX

SUNY BROCKPORT

3 2815 00837 5753

RC 66 .J4613 2001

Jenicek, Milos, 1935-

Clinical case reporting in
evidence-based medicine

DATE DUE

DEC 0 4 2002		
OCT 0 7 2003		

GAYLORD PRINTED IN U.S.A.

DRAKE MEMORIAL LIBRARY
WITHDRAWN
THE COLLEGE AT BROCKPORT